Renal Cookbook

The Best Low Sodium, Potassium, and Phosphorous Recipes to Control Kidney Disease and Improve your Health

Olivia Dixon

inattention, use, or misuse of the information in question by the reader will render any resulting actions solely under their purview. There are no scenarios in which the publisher or the original author of this work can be in any fashion deemed liable for any hardship or damages that may befall them after undertaking information described herein.

Additionally, the information in the following pages is intended only for informational purposes and should thus be thought of as universal. As befitting its nature, it is presented without assurance regarding its prolonged validity or interim quality. Trademarks that are mentioned are done without written consent and can in no way be considered an endorsement from the trademark holder.

TABLE OF CONTENT

Introduction

kidney disease is becoming more prevalent and so we need to learn as much about it as we can. The more we educate ourselves, the more we can do to take care of this important bodily system. If you've been diagnosed with chronic kidney disease (CKD), education can empower you to most effectively and purposefully manage the disease. Once you have a full understanding of what chronic kidney disease is, you can begin to take charge of your evolving health needs.

Our kidneys do powerful things to keep our bodies in balance. When everything is working properly, the kidneys do many important jobs such as:

- Filtering waste materials from the blood.
- Removing extra fluid, or water, from the body.
- Releasing hormones that help manage blood pressure.
- Stimulating bone marrow to make red blood cells.
- Making an active form of vitamin D that promotes strong, healthy bones.

There are many causes of kidney disease, including physical injury or disorders that can damage the kidneys, but the two leading causes of kidney diseases are diabetes and high blood pressure. These underlying conditions also put people at risk of developing cardiovascular disease. Early treatment may not only slow down the progression of the disease but also reduce your risk of developing heart disease or stroke.

Kidney disease can affect anyone at any age.

We have established the importance of a renal diet and why you should include it in your lifestyle. Most people assume that it's difficult to follow the renal diet, but it's easier than you think. To get the best results (improved kidney function, reduced dialysis risk), it is important to learn more about kidney disease diet. When you learn what to eat and avoid, it becomes a lot easier to adjust your eating habits. So, before we start cooking some delicious foods, we will go through the list of foods you should eat and avoid managing kidney disease.

It's important to repeat that diet restrictions vary according to the stage of kidney disease. Renal diet usually involves limiting potassium and sodium consumption to 2000 mg a day and lowering phosphorus intake to 1000 mg per day.

Foods to Eat

When it comes to a renal diet, you must opt for low sodium, potassium, phosphorus, and protein.

- *Onions*: sodium-free flavor for renal diet.
- *Egg whites*
- *Cauliflower:* anti-inflammatory properties, abundant in vitamin C, vitamin K, and folate. *Blueberries*: nutrient-rich and abundant in antioxidants that decrease the risk of diabetes, heart disease, and cognitive decline.

- *Turnip*: excellent replacement for high-potassium vegetables such as potatoes.
- *Cabbage*: a source of vitamin K, vitamin C, and B-complex vitamins.
- *Sea bass*: high-quality protein and a good source of Omega-3 fatty acids.
- *Garlic*: a delicious alternative to salt.
- *Buckwheat*: nutritious, rich in fiber, magnesium, iron, and B vitamins.
- *Olive oil*: phosphorus-free.
- *Bulgur*: kidney-friendly alternative to whole grains.
- *Bell peppers:* low in potassium.
- *Arugula*: nutrient-dense green vegetable low in potassium.
- *Red grapes*: rich in vitamin C and other valuable nutrients.
- *Macadamia nuts*: low in phosphorus.
- *Radish:* low in potassium and phosphorus.
- *Pineapple*: low potassium content.
- *Cranberries*
- *Shiitake mushrooms*
- *Apples*

Foods to Avoid

To follow the renal diet that will support kidney function and not disrupt it, you may want to avoid consuming the following foods:

- *Avocado*
- *Whole-wheat bread*
- Brown rice: high in potassium and phosphorus.
- Bananas: abundant in potassium.
- *Oranges*: a rich source of potassium.
- *Processed meat*: contain high amounts of salt.
- *Olives, pickles, and relish*
- *Apricots*
- *Potatoes*
- *Tomatoes*
- *Instant, packaged, and premade meals*
- *Spinach*: contain high amounts of potassium.
- *Prunes, raisins, and dates*

Fluids and Juices for Healthy Kidneys

Management of kidney disease also requires paying attention to fluid intake and the things you drink. For example, you should avoid soda, especially dark-colored cola. But, here are some drinks you should include in your lifestyle:

- *Cranberry juice*: beneficial for urinary and kidney health.

- *Lemon-* and lime-based or other citrus juice
- *Water*
- *Stinging nettle tea*: antioxidant-rich, reduces inflammation.

Breakfast Recipes

Spring Muffin

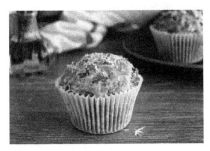

Preparation Time: 10 minutes **Cooking Time:** 35 Minutes

Servings:12

Ingredients:

- ✓ 1 tablespoon olive oil
- ✓ 1 cup red bell pepper, chopped
- ✓ 1 green bell pepper, chopped
- ✓ 1 cup onion, chopped
- ✓ 2 cup spinach, chopped
- ✓ 2 cloves of garlic
- ✓ 1 cup mushrooms, chopped
- ✓ 4 eggs

Directions:

1. Preheat oven to 350°F.
2. Heat oil in a pan.
3. Add peppers, onion, and cook.
4. Place spinach, garlic, and mushrooms and cook for two more minutes.

5   In a mixing bowl, add the eggs and blend.

6   Stir in cooked vegetables.

7   Spread the batter into the muffin tray.

8   Bake for about 20 minutes.

9   Serve and enjoy!

Nutrition:

Calories 54 Carbohydrates 3 g Protein 4 g Sodium 38 mg

Egg White Scramble

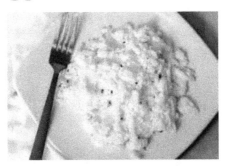

Preparation Time: 10 minutes **Cooking Time:** 6 minutes

Servings: 4

Ingredients:

- ✓ 1 teaspoon almond butter
- ✓ 4 egg whites
- ✓ ¼ teaspoon salt
- ✓ ½ teaspoon paprika
- ✓ 2 tablespoons heavy cream

Directions:

1. Whisk the egg whites gently and add heavy cream.
2. Put the almond butter in the skillet and melt it.
3. Then add egg white mixture.
4. Sprinkle it with salt and cook for 2 minutes over medium heat.
5. After this, scramble the egg whites with the fork or spatula's help and sprinkle with paprika.
6. Cook the scrambled egg whites for 3 minutes more.

17

7   Transfer the meal to the serving plates.

Nutrition:

Calories: 68 Fat: 5.1 g Fiber: 0.5 g Carbs: 1.3 g Protein: 4.6 g

Blackberry Pudding

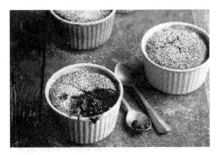

Preparation time: 45 minutes **Cooking time:** 5 minutes

Servings: 2

Ingredients:

- ✓ ¼ cup chia seeds
- ✓ ½ cup blackberries, fresh
- ✓ 1 teaspoon liquid sweetener
- ✓ 1 cup coconut milk, full fat and unsweetened
- ✓ 1 teaspoon vanilla extract

Directions:

1. Take the vanilla, liquid sweetener and coconut milk and add to blender.
2. Process until thick.
3. Add blackberries and process until smooth.
4. Divide the mixture between cups and chill for 30 minutes. Serve and enjoy!

Nutrition:

Calories: 437 Fat: 38g Carbohydrates: 8g Protein: 8g

Vanilla Cereals

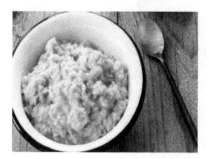

Preparation time: 10 minutes **Cooking time:** 25 minutes

Servings: 4

Ingredients:

- ✓ 2¼ cups water
- ✓ 1¼ cups vanilla rice milk
- ✓ 6 tablespoons uncooked bulgur
- ✓ 1 tablespoon uncooked whole buckwheat
- ✓ 1 cup apple, peeled and sliced
- ✓ 6 tablespoons plain uncooked couscous
- ✓ ½ teaspoon ground cinnamon

Directions:

1   Heat the water and the rice milk in a pan over medium-high heat.
2   Add the bulgur, buckwheat, and apple.
3   Cook for about 25 minutes, stirring occasionally.
4   Remove the saucepan from the heat.
5   Let the saucepan stand for 10 minutes.

6   Serve and enjoy!

Calories 172 Fat 1 g Cholesterol 0 mg Carbohydrates 35 g
Sugar 7 g Fiber 4 g Protein 4 g Sodium 34 mg

Egg White and Pepper Omelet

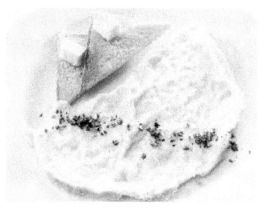

Preparation time: 5 minutes **Cooking time:** 5 minutes

Servings: 2

Ingredients:

- ✓ 4 egg whites, lightly beaten
- ✓ 1 red bell pepper, diced
- ✓ 1 tsp. of paprika
- ✓ 2 tbsp. of olive oil
- ✓ ½ tsp. of salt Pepper

Directions:

1 In a shallow pan (around 8 inches), heat the olive oil and sauté the bell peppers until softened.
2 Add the egg whites and the paprika, fold the edges into the fluid center with a spatula and let the omelet cook until eggs are fully opaque and solid.
3 Season with salt and pepper.

Nutrition:

Calories: 165 Carbohydrate: 3.8 g Protein: 9.2 g Sodium: 797 mg Potassium: 193 mg Phosphorus: 202.5 mg Dietary Fiber: 0.7 g Fat: 15.22 g

Turkey Pinwheels

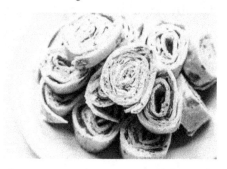

Preparation time: 10 minutes **Cooking time:** 17 minutes

Servings: 6

Ingredients:

- ✓ 6 toothpicks
- ✓ 8 oz. spring mix salad greens
- ✓ 1 ten-inch tortilla
- ✓ 2 oz. thinly sliced deli turkey
- ✓ 9 tsp. whipped cream cheese
- ✓ 1 red bell pepper, roasted

Directions:

1 Cut the red bell pepper into ten strips about ¼ -inch thick. Spread the whipped cream cheese on the tortilla evenly.

2 Add the salad greens to create a base layer and then lay the turkey on top of it.

3 Space out the red bell pepper strips on top of the turkey.

4 Tuck the end and begin rolling the tortilla inward.

24

5 Use the toothpicks to hold the roll into place and cut it into six pieces.

6 Serve with the swirl facing upward.

Nutrition:

Calories: 206 Fats: 9 g Carbs: 21 g Protein: 9 g Sodium: 533 mg Potassium: 145 mg Phosphorus: 47 mg

Apple and Cinnamon French toast Strata

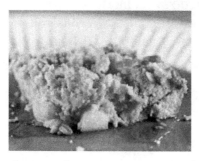

Preparation time: 2 hr 15 minutes **Cooking time:** 50 minutes

Servings: 12

Ingredients:

- ✓ 2 apples peeled, diced
- ✓ 1-pound cinnamon and raisin loaf, diced
- ✓ 1 teaspoon ground cinnamon
- ✓ ¼ cup pancake syrup
- ✓ 6 tablespoons unsalted butter, melted
- ✓ 1 ¼ cup half-and-half creamer
- ✓ 8 ounces cream cheese, softened and cubed
- ✓ 8 large eggs
- ✓ 1 ¼ cup almond milk, unsweetened

Directions:

1   Take a nine 13 inches baking dish, grease it with oil, then arrange half of the bread cubes on the bottom and

26

scatter cream cheese evenly on the top.

2   Top cream cheese with the apple, sprinkle with cinnamon and then top with remaining bread cubes.

3   Crack eggs in a large bowl, add pancake syrup, butter, milk, and creamer, whisk until combined, pour this mixture evenly in the prepared casserole, cover it with plastic wrap, and then keep the casserole dish in the refrigerator for 2 hours.

4   When ready to cook, switch on the oven, set it to 325°F, and preheat.

5   Then uncover casserole, bake for 50 minutes.

6   Drizzle with more pancake syrup and then serve.

Nutrition:

Calories 324, Fat 20 g, Protein 9 g, Carbohydrates 27 g, Fiber 1.8 g

Tofu and Mushroom Scramble

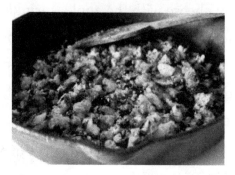

Preparation time: 5 minutes **Cooking time:** 10 minutes

Servings: 2

Ingredients:

- ✓ ½ cup of sliced white mushrooms
- ✓ ⅓ cup of medium-firm tofu, crumbled
- ✓ 1 tbsp. of chopped shallots
- ✓ ⅓ tsp. of turmeric 1 tsp. of cumin
- ✓ ⅓ tsp. of smoked paprika
- ✓ ½ tsp. of garlic salt Pepper
- ✓ 3 tbsp. of vegetable oil

Directions:

1 Heat the oil frying pan, set it on a medium, and sauté the sliced mushrooms with the shallots until softened (around 3–4 minutes) over medium to high heat.

2 Add the tofu pieces and toss in the spices and the garlic salt. Toss lightly until tofu and mushrooms are nicely combined.

Nutrition:

Calories: 220 Carbohydrate: 2.59 g Protein: 3.2 g Sodium: 288 mg Potassium: 133.5 mg Phosphorus: 68.5 mg Dietary Fiber: 1.7 g Fat: 23.7 g

Cauliflower Rice and Coconut

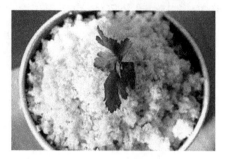

Preparation time: 20 minutes **Cooking time:** 30 minutes

Servings: 4

Ingredients:

- ✓ 3 cups cauliflower, riced
- ✓ 2/3 cups full-fat coconut milk
- ✓ 1–2 tsp. sriracha
- ✓ ¼–½ tsp. onion powder
- ✓ Salt as needed Fresh basil for garnish

Directions:

1   Take a pan and place it over medium-low heat.
2   Add all the ingredients and stir them until fully combined. Cook for about 5–10 minutes, making sure that the lid is on. Remove the lid and keep cooking until there's no excess liquid. Once the rice is soft and creamy, enjoy it!

Nutrition:

Calories: 95 Fats: 7 g Carbs: 4 g Protein: 1 g

Avocado Toast with Egg

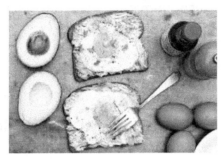

Preparation time: 10 minutes **Cooking time:** 5 minutes

Servings: 2

Ingredients:

- ✓ ½ of a medium avocado, pitted and sliced
- ✓ tablespoon parsley, chopped
- ✓ ¼ teaspoon ground black pepper
- ✓ 1/8 teaspoon salt
- ✓ tablespoon lime juice
- ✓ tablespoons feta cheese, crumbled
- ✓ eggs
- ✓ slices of whole-grain bread, toasted

Directions:

1 Transfer avocado flesh to a medium bowl, mash with a fork and then stir in salt and lime juice.

2 Put the avocado mixture evenly onto each piece of toast, then take a skillet pan, spray it with oil and hot, crack eggs into it and cook to the desired level.

3 Distribute eggs onto the toast, top each piece of toast with ½ tablespoon parsley, one tablespoon cheese, and 1/8 teaspoon ground black pepper.

4 Serve straight away.

Nutrition:

Calories 225, Fat 13 g, Protein 12 g, Carbohydrates15 g, Fiber 4

Egg Fried Rice

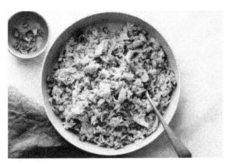

Preparation time: 10 minutes **Cooking time:** 20 minutes

Servings: 6

Ingredients:

- ✓ 1 tablespoon of olive oil
- ✓ 1 tablespoon of grated peeled fresh ginger
- ✓ 1 teaspoon of minced garlic
- ✓ 1 cup of chopped carrots
- ✓ 1 scallion, white and green parts, chopped
- ✓ 2 tablespoons of chopped fresh cilantro
- ✓ cups of cooked rice
- ✓ 1 tablespoon of low-sodium soy sauce
- ✓ 4 eggs, beaten

Directions:

1 Heat the olive oil.

2 Add the ginger and garlic, and sauté until softened, about 3 minutes.

3 Add the carrots, scallion, and cilantro, and sauté until

tender, about 5 minutes.

4   Stir in the rice and soy sauce, and sauté until the rice is heated over 5 minutes.

5   Move the rice over to one side of the skillet, and pour the eggs into the space.

6   Scramble the eggs, then mix them into the rice.

7   Serve hot.

8   Low-sodium tip: Soy sauces, even low-sodium versions, are very salty. If you have the time, making your substitution sauce is simple and effective, even if it does not taste quite the same. Many versions of this diet-friendly sauce are online, with ingredients like vinegar, molasses, garlic, and herbs.

Nutrition:

Calories: 204 Total fat: 6 g Saturated fat: 1 g Cholesterol: 141 mg Sodium: 223 mg Carbohydrates: 29 g Fiber: 1 g Phosphorus: 120 mg Potassium: 147 mg Protein: 8 g

Breakfast Burrito

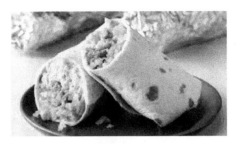

Preparation time: 15 minutes **Cooking time:** 3 minutes

Servings: 2

Ingredients:

- ✓ 3 tablespoons green chilies, diced
- ✓ ½ teaspoon hot pepper sauce
- ✓ ¼ teaspoon ground cumin
- ✓ eggs
- ✓ 2 flour tortillas, burrito size

Directions:

1. Take a medium-sized skillet pan, place it over medium heat, grease it with oil, and let it get hot.
2. Crack eggs in a bowl, add chilies, hot sauce, and cumin, whisk until combined, then cook for 2 minutes, or until eggs have been cooked to the desired level.
3. Meanwhile, heat the tortillas by microwaving
4. m for 20 seconds until hot.
5. When eggs have cooked, distribute evenly between hot tortillas, and roll it up like a burrito.

6   Serve straight away.

Nutrition:

Calories 366, Fat 18 g, Protein 18 g, Carbohydrates 33 g, Fiber 2.5 g

Grandma's Pancake Special

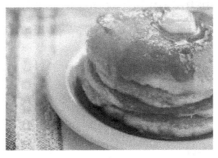

Preparation time: 5 minutes **Cooking time:** 10 minutes

Servings: 3

Ingredients:

- ✓ 1 tbsp. oil
- ✓ 1 cup milk
- ✓ 1 egg
- ✓ 2 tsp. sodium-free baking powder
- ✓ 2 tbsp. sugar
- ✓ 1 ¼ cups flour

Directions:

1 Mix together all the dry ingredients such as the flour, sugar, and baking powder.

2 Combine the oil, milk, and egg in another bowl. Once done, add them all to the flour mixture.

3 Make sure that as you stir the mixture, you blend them together until slightly lumpy.

4 In a hot, greased griddle, pour in at least ¼ cup of the

batter to make each pancake.

5   To cook, ensure that the bottom is a bit brown, then turn and cook the other side as well.

Nutrition:

Calories: 167 Carbs: 50 g Protein: 11 g Fats: 11 g Phosphorus: 176 mg Potassium: 215 mg Sodium: 70 mg

Chocolate Coconut Porridge

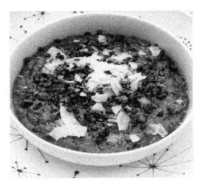

Preparation time: 5 minutes **Cooking time:** 10 minutes

Servings: 1

Ingredients:

- ✓ 2 tablespoons cornstarch
- ✓ 2 tablespoons of grated coconut
- ✓ glasses of milk
- ✓ 2 large spoons of chocolate powder

Directions:

1. First, put the milk and two tablespoons cornstarch.
2. Bring to the heat and add the well-grated coconut.
3. Finally, put the chocolate.
4. Stir until desired consistency.

Nutrition:

Calories 79,Fat 2 g,Protein 4 g,Carbohydrates 10 g,Fiber 0.2 g

Pineapple Bread

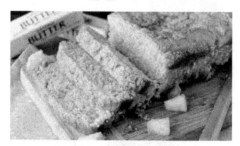

Preparation time: 25 minutes **Cooking time:** 1 hr

Servings: 10

Ingredients:

- ✓ 1/3 cup Swerver
- ✓ 1/3 cup butter, unsalted
- ✓ 2 eggs
- ✓ 2 cups flour
- ✓ 3 tsp. baking powder
- ✓ 1 cup pineapple, undrained
- ✓ cherries, chopped

Directions:

1 Whisk the Swerver with the butter in a mixer until fluffy.
2 Stir in the eggs, then beat again.
3 Add the baking powder and flour, then mix well until smooth. Fold in the cherries and pineapple.
4 Spread this cherry-pineapple batter in a 9x5-inch baking pan.

5   Bake the pineapple batter for 1 hour at 350°F.

6   Slice the bread and serve.

Nutrition:

Calories: 197 Fats: 7.2 g Sodium: 85 mg Fiber: 1.1 g Sugars 3 g

Protein 4 g Calcium: 79 mg Phosphorous: 316 mg Potassium:

227 mg

Italian Breakfast Frittata

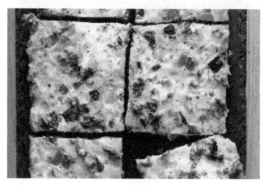

Preparation time: 15 minutes **Cooking time:** 40 minutes

Servings: 4

Ingredients:

- ✓ 2 cups egg whites
- ✓ ½ cup mozzarella cheese, shredded
- ✓ 1 cup cottage cheese, crumbled
- ✓ ¼ cup fresh basil, sliced
- ✓ ½ cup roasted red peppers, sliced
- ✓ Pepper Salt

Directions:

1 Preheat the oven to 375°F.

2 Add all the ingredients into the large bowl and whisk well to combine.

3 Pour the frittata mixture into the baking dish and bake for 45 minutes.

4 Slice and serve.

Nutrition:

Calories: 131 Fats: 2 g Carbs: 5 g Sugar: 2 g Protein: 22 g
Cholesterol: 6 mg

Chocolate & Banana Muffins

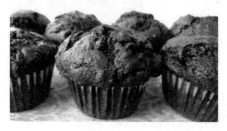

Preparation time: 25 minutes **Cooking time:** 15 minutes

Servings: 12

Ingredients:

- ✓ 2 large softened bananas
- ✓ 1 large egg
- ✓ 1/3 cup light brown sugar
- ✓ ¼ cup olive oil
- ✓ 2 tablespoons plain yogurt
- ✓ 1 teaspoon vanilla extract
- ✓ 1 cup unbleached, all-purpose flour
- ✓ ¼ teaspoon of sea salt
- ✓ ½ teaspoon baking soda
- ✓ ¼ teaspoon nutmeg
- ✓ 1/3 cup almonds, sliced
- ✓ 2/3 cup dark chocolate chip

Directions:

1 Preheat the oven to 350°F.

2 Put a muffin tray with cooking spray and set aside.

3   In a mixing bowl, add bananas, egg, sugar, and oil.

4   Put yogurt and vanilla and mix with a fork until smooth.

5   Add the flour ¼ cup at a time, with salt and baking soda in between additions.

6   Stir well.

7   Combine almonds and chocolate chips.

8   Bake for about 12 minutes.

9   Serve and enjoy!

Nutrition:

Calories 148 Fat 7 g Cholesterol 15 mg Carbohydrates 19 g Sugar 8 g Fiber 1 g Protein 3 g Sodium 111 mg Calcium 22 mg Phosphorus 45 mg Potassium 140 mg

Arugula Eggs with Chili Peppers

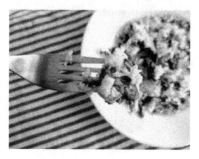

Preparation time: 10 minutes **Cooking time:** 5 minutes

Servings: 4

Ingredients:

- ✓ 2 cups arugula, chopped
- ✓ 3 eggs, beaten
- ✓ ½ chili pepper, chopped
- ✓ 1 tablespoon butter
- ✓ 1 oz Parmesan, grated

Directions:

1. Toss butter in the skillet and melt it.
2. Add arugula and sauté it over medium heat for 5 minutes. Stir it from time to time.
3. Meanwhile, mix up together Parmesan, chili pepper, and eggs. Pour the egg mixture over the arugula and scramble well.
4. Cook the breakfast for 5 minutes more over medium heat.

Nutrition:

Calories: 98 Fat: 7.8 g Fiber: 0.2 g Carbs: 0.9 g Protein: 6.7 g

Green lettuce Bacon Breakfast Bake

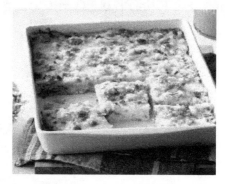

Preparation time: 15 minutes **Cooking time:** 45 minutes

Servings: 6

Ingredients:

- ✓ eggs
- ✓ 3 cups baby green lettuce, chopped
- ✓ 1 tbsp. olive oil
- ✓ bacon slices, cooked and chopped
- ✓ 2 red bell peppers, sliced
- ✓ 2 tbsp. chives, chopped
- ✓ Pepper Salt
- ✓ Cooking spray

Directions:

1 Preheat the oven to 350°F.
2 Spray a baking dish with the cooking spray and set it aside. Heat the oil in a pan. 4. Add the green lettuce and cook until the green lettuce is wilted.

48

3 In a mixing bowl, whisk the eggs and salt. Add the green lettuce and chives and stir well.

4 Pour the egg mixture into the baking dish.

5 Top with the red bell peppers and bacon and bake for 45 minutes.

6 Serve and enjoy.

Nutrition:

Calories: 273 Fat: 20.4 g Carbs: 3.1 g Sugar: 1.7 g Protein: 19.4 g Cholesterol: 301 mg

Panzanella Salad

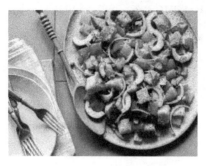

Preparation time: 12 minutes **Cooking time:** 5 minutes

Servings: 4

Ingredients:

- ✓ 2 cucumbers, chopped
- ✓ 1 red onion, sliced
- ✓ 2 red bell peppers, chopped
- ✓ ¼ cup fresh cilantro, chopped
- ✓ 1 tablespoon capers
- ✓ 1 oz whole-grain bread, chopped
- ✓ 1 tablespoon canola oil
- ✓ ½ teaspoon minced garlic
- ✓ 1 tablespoon Dijon mustard
- ✓ 1 teaspoon olive oil
- ✓ 1 teaspoon lime juice

Directions:

1　Pour canola oil into the skillet and bring it to boil.

2　Add chopped bread and roast it until crunchy (3-5

minutes). Meanwhile, in the salad bowl, combine sliced red onion, cucumbers, bell peppers, cilantro, capers, and mix up gently. Make the dressing: mix up together lime juice, olive oil, Dijon mustard, and minced garlic.

3   Transfer the dressing over the salad and stir it directly before serving.

Nutrition:

Calories: 136 Fat: 5.7 g Fiber: 4.1 g Carbs: 20.2 g Protein: 4.1 g

Vegetable Recipes

Carrot-Apple Casserole

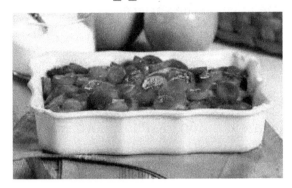

Preparation time: 20 minutes **Cooking time:** 50 minutes

Servings: 6

Ingredients:

- ✓ large carrots, peeled and sliced
- ✓ large apples, peeled and sliced
- ✓ 3 tbsps. Butter
- ✓ ½ cup apple juice
- ✓ tbsps. all-purpose flour
- ✓ 2 tbsps. brown sugar
- ✓ ½ tsp ground nutmeg

Directions:

1. Preheat oven to 350°F.
2. Let the carrots boil for 5 minutes or until tender. Drain. Arrange the carrots and apples in a large casserole dish.
3. Mix the flour, brown sugar, and nutmeg in a small bowl.
4. Rub in the butter to make a crumb topping.

5 Sprinkle the crumb over the carrots and apples, then pour the juice on the surface.

6 Bake until bubbling and golden brown.

Nutrition:

Calories: 245 Fats: 6 g Carbs: 49 g Protein: 1 g Sodium: 91 mg Potassium: 169 mg Phosphorous: 17 mg

Fast Cabbage Cakes

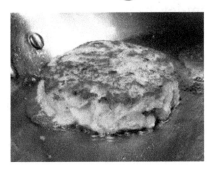

Preparation time: 10 minutes **Cooking time:** 15 minutes

Servings: 2

Ingredients:

- ✓ 1 cup cauliflower, shredded
- ✓ 1 egg, beaten
- ✓ 1 teaspoon salt
- ✓ 1 teaspoon ground black pepper
- ✓ 1 tablespoon almond flour
- ✓ 1 teaspoon olive oil

Directions:

1. Blend the shredded cabbage in the blender until you get cabbage rice.
2. Then, mix up cabbage rice with the egg, salt, ground black pepper, and almond flour.
3. Pour olive oil into the skillet and preheat it.
4. Then make the small cakes with the help of 2 spoons and place them in the hot oil.

5 Roast the cabbage cakes for 4 minutes from each side over medium-low heat.

6 It is recommended to use a non-stick skillet.

Nutrition:

Calories 227, Fat 18.6, Fiber 4.5, Carbs 9.5, Protein 9.9

Zucchini Bowl

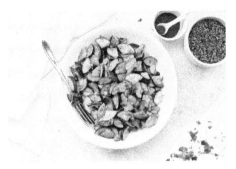

Preparation time: 20 minutes **Cooking time:** 15 minutes

Servings: 2

Ingredients:

- ✓ 1 onion, chopped
- ✓ 3 zucchini, cut into medium chunks
- ✓ 2 tablespoons coconut milk
- ✓ garlic cloves, minced
- ✓ 3 cups chicken stock
- ✓ 2 tablespoons coconut oil
- ✓ Pinch of salt
- ✓ Black pepper to taste

Directions:

1. Take a pot and place it over medium heat.
2. Add oil and let it heat up.
3. Add zucchini, garlic, onion, and stir.
4. Cook for 5 minutes.
5. Add stock, salt, pepper, and stir.

6 Bring to a boil and lower down the heat.

7 Simmer for 20 minutes.

8 Remove heat and add coconut milk.

9 Use an immersion blender until smooth.

10 Ladle into soup bowls and serve Enjoy!

Nutrition:

Calories: 160 Fat: 2 g Carbohydrates: 4 g Protein: 7 g

Cauliflower Rice

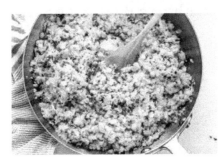

Preparation time: 5 minutes **Cooking time:** 15 minutes

Servings: 1

Ingredients:

- ✓ 1 small head cauliflower cut into florets
- ✓ 1 tbsp. butter
- ✓ ¼ tsp. black pepper
- ✓ ¼ tsp. garlic powder
- ✓ ¼ tsp. salt-free herb seasoning blend

Directions:

1. Blitz the cauliflower pieces in a food processor until it has a grain- like consistency.
2. Melt the butter in a saucepan and add spices.
3. Add the cauliflower rice grains and cook over low-medium heat for approximately 10 minutes.
4. Use a fork to fluff the rice before serving.
5. Serve as an alternative to rice with curries, stews, and starch to accompany meat and fish dishes.

Nutrition:

Calories: 47 Carbs: 4 g Protein: 1 g Sodium: 300 mg

Potassium: 206 mg Phosphorous: 31 mg

Mushroom Tacos

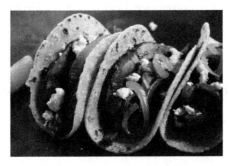

Preparation time: 10 minutes **Cooking time:** 15 minutes

Servings: 6

Ingredients:

- ✓ collard greens leave
- ✓ 2 cups mushrooms, chopped
- ✓ 1 white onion, diced
- ✓ 1 tablespoon Taco seasoning
- ✓ 1 tablespoon coconut oil
- ✓ ½ teaspoon salt
- ✓ ¼ cup fresh parsley
- ✓ 1 tablespoon mayonnaise

Directions:

1 Put the coconut oil in the skillet and melt it.

2 Add chopped mushrooms and diced onion. Mix up the ingredients.

3 Close the lid and cook them for 10 minutes.

4 After this, sprinkle the vegetables with Taco seasoning,

salt, and add fresh parsley.

5 Mix up the mixture and cook for 5 minutes more.

6 Then add mayonnaise and stir well.

7 Chill the mushroom mixture a little.

8 Fill the collard green leaves with the mushroom mixture and fold up them.

Nutrition:

Calories 52, fat 3.3, fiber 1.2, carbs 5.1, protein 1.4

Vegetable Biryani

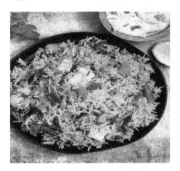

Preparation time: 20 minutes **Cooking time:** 15 minutes

Servings: 4

Ingredients:

- ✓ 2 tablespoons olive oil
- ✓ 1 onion, diced
- ✓ garlic cloves, minced
- ✓ 1 tablespoon peeled and grated fresh ginger root
- ✓ 1 cup carrot, grated
- ✓ 2 cups chopped cauliflower
- ✓ 1 cup frozen baby peas, thawed and drained
- ✓ 2 teaspoons curry powder
- ✓ 1 cup low-sodium vegetable broth
- ✓ cups frozen cooked rice

Directions:

1 In a large skillet, heat the olive oil over medium heat.

2 Add the onion, garlic, and ginger root and sauté, frequently stirring until tender-crisp, 2 minutes.

3   Add the carrot, cauliflower, peas, and curry powder and cook for 2 minutes longer.

4   Stir in the vegetable broth and bring to a simmer. Reduce the heat to low, partially cover the skillet, and simmer for 6 to 7 minutes or until the vegetables are tender.

5   Meanwhile, heat the rice as directed on the package.

6   Stir the rice into the vegetable mixture and serve.

Nutrition:

Calories: 378 Total Fat: 16 g Saturated Fat: 2 g Cholesterol: 0 mg Sodium: 113 mg Total Carbs: 53 g Fiber: 7 g Sugar: 6 g Protein: 8 g

Pesto Pasta Salad

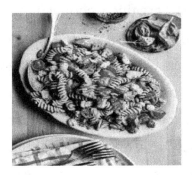

Preparation time: 15 minutes **Cooking time:** 15 minutes

Servings: 4

Ingredients:

- ✓ 1 cup fresh basil leaves
- ✓ ½ cup packed fresh flat-leaf parsley leaves
- ✓ ½ cup arugula, chopped
- ✓ 2 tbsps. Parmesan cheese, grated
- ✓ ¼ cup extra-virgin olive oil
- ✓ 2 tbsps. Mayonnaise
- ✓ 2 tbsps. water
- ✓ oz. whole wheat rotini pasta
- ✓ 1 red bell pepper, chopped
- ✓ 1 medium yellow summer squash, sliced
- ✓ 1 cup baby peas, frozen

Directions:

1 Boil water in a large pot.

2 Meanwhile, combine the basil, parsley, arugula, cheese,

and olive oil in a blender or food processor. Process until the herbs are finely chopped. Add the mayonnaise and water, then process again. Set aside.

3   Prepare the pasta to the pot of boiling water; cook according to package directions, about 8 to 9 minutes.

4   Combine the pesto, pasta, bell pepper, squash, and peas in a large bowl and toss gently, adding enough reserved pasta cooking liquid to make a sauce on the salad. Serve immediately or cover and chill, then serve.

5   Cover and store it in the refrigerator for up to 3 days.

Nutrition:

Calories: 378 Fats: 24 g Carbs: 35 g Protein: 9 g Sodium: 163 mg Potassium: 472 mg Phosphorus: 213 mg

Vegetable Masala

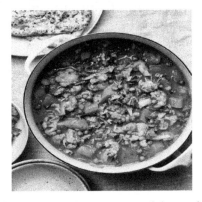

Preparation time: 15 minutes **Cooking time:** 15 minutes

Servings: 4

Ingredients:

- ✓ 2 cups green beans, chopped
- ✓ 1 cup white mushroom, chopped
- ✓ ¾ cup tomatoes, crushed
- ✓ 1 teaspoon minced garlic
- ✓ 1 teaspoon minced ginger
- ✓ 1 teaspoon chili flakes
- ✓ 1 tablespoon gram masala
- ✓ 1 tablespoon olive oil
- ✓ 1 teaspoon salt

Directions:

1 Line the tray with parchment and preheat the oven to 360F. Place the green beans and mushrooms in the tray.

2   Sprinkle the vegetables with crushed tomatoes, minced garlic and ginger, chili flakes, masala, olive oil, and salt.

3   Mix up well and transfer in the oven.

4   Cook vegetable masala for 18 minutes.

Nutrition:

Calories 60, Fat 30.7, Fiber 2.5, Carbs 6.4, Protein 2

Roasted Veggie Sandwiches

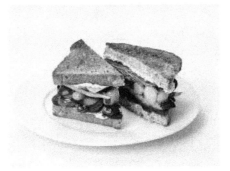

Preparation time: 15 minutes **Cooking time:** 35 minutes

Servings: 6

Ingredients:

- ✓ 3 peppers, assorted colors, sliced
- ✓ 1 cup of sliced yellow summer squash
- ✓ 1 red onion, sliced 2 tablespoons of extra-virgin olive oil
- ✓ 2 tablespoons of balsamic vinegar
- ✓ ⅛ teaspoon of salt
- ✓ ⅛ teaspoon of freshly ground black pepper
- ✓ large whole-wheat pita breads, halved

Directions:

1 Preheat the oven to 400°F.

2 Prepare a parchment paper and line it with a rimmed baking sheet. Spread the bell peppers, squash, and onion on the prepared baking sheet. Sprinkle with the olive oil, vinegar, salt, and pepper.

3 Roast for 30 to 40 minutes, turning the vegetables with a spatula once during cooking until they are tender and light golden brown.

4 Pile the vegetables into the pieces of pita bread and serve.

Nutrition:

Calories: 182 Total Fat: 5 g Saturated Fat: 1 g Sodium: 234 mg Phosphorus: 106 mg Potassium: 289 mg Carbohydrates: 31 g Fiber: 4 g Protein: 5 g Sugar: 6 g

Jicama Noodles

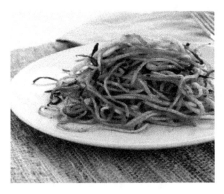

Preparation time: 15 minutes **Cooking time:** 5 minutes

Servings: 6

Ingredients:

- ✓ 1 lb. jicama, peeled
- ✓ 2 tbsps. Butter
- ✓ 1 tsp. chili flakes
- ✓ 1 tsp. salt
- ✓ ¾ cup water

Directions:

1 Spiralize the jicama with the help of a spiralizer and place in jicama spirals in the saucepan.

2 Add the butter, chili flakes, and salt.

3 Then add the water and preheat the ingredients until the butter is melted.

4 Mix up it well.

5 Close the lid and cook the noodles for 4 minutes over

medium heat.

6   Stir the jicama noodles well before transferring them to the serving plates.

Nutrition:

Calories:63 Fats: 3.9 g Fiber: 3.7 g Carbs: 6.7 g Protein: 0.6 g

Crack Slaw

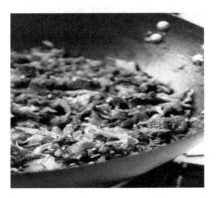

Preparation time: 15 minutes **Cooking time:** 10 minutes

Servings: 6

Ingredients:

- ✓ 1 cup cauliflower rice
- ✓ 1 teaspoon tahini paste
- ✓ 1 teaspoon sesame seeds
- ✓ 1 tablespoon lemon juice
- ✓ 1 teaspoon olive oil
- ✓ 1 teaspoon butter
- ✓ ½ teaspoon salt
- ✓ 2 cups coleslaw

Directions:

1. Toss the butter in the skillet and melt it.
2. Add cauliflower rice and sprinkle it with tahini paste.
3. Mix up the vegetables and cook them for 10 minutes over medium heat. Stir them from time to time.

4 When the cauliflower is cooked, transfer it to the big plate. Add coleslaw and stir gently.

5 Then sprinkle the salad with sesame seeds, lemon juice, olive oil, and salt.

6 Mix up well.

Nutrition:

Nutrition: calories 76, fat 5.8, fiber 0.6, carbs 6, protein 1.1

Spicy Corn and Rice Burritos

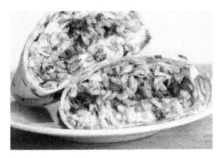

Preparation time: 15 minutes **Cooking time:** 20 minutes

Servings: 4

Ingredients:

- ✓ tablespoons of extra-virgin olive oil, divided
- ✓ 1 (10-ounce) package of frozen cooked rice 1
- ✓ ½ cups of frozen yellow corn
- ✓ 1 tablespoon of chili powder
- ✓ 1 cup of shredded pepper jack cheese
- ✓ large or 6 small corn tortillas

Directions:

1. Put the skillet in over medium heat and put 2 tablespoons of olive oil. Add the rice, corn, and chili powder and cook for 4 to 6 minutes, or until the ingredients are hot.

2. Transfer the ingredients from the pan into a medium bowl. Let cool for 15 minutes.

3. Stir the cheese into the rice mixture.

4. Heat the tortillas using the directions from the package

to make them pliable. Fill the corn tortillas with the rice mixture, then roll them up.

5   At this point, you can serve them as is, or you can fry them first. Heat the remaining tablespoon of olive oil in a large skillet.

6   Fry the burritos, seam-side down at first, turning once, until they are brown and crisp, about 4 to 6 minutes per side, then serve.

Nutrition:

Calories: 386 Total Fat: 21 g Saturated Fat: 7 g Sodium: 510 mg Phosphorus: 304 mg Potassium: 282 mg Carbohydrates: 41 g Fiber: 4 g Protein: 11 g Sugar: 2 g

Shrimp Bruschetta

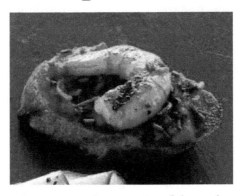

Preparation time: 15 minutes **Cooking time:** 15 minutes

Servings: 4

Ingredients:

- ✓ 13 oz. shrimps, peeled
- ✓ 1 tbsp. tomato sauce
- ✓ ½ tsp. Splenda
- ✓ ¼ tsp. garlic powder
- ✓ 1 tsp. fresh parsley, chopped
- ✓ ½ tsp. olive oil
- ✓ 1 tsp. lemon juice
- ✓ whole-grain bread slices
- ✓ 1 cup water

Directions:

1 In the saucepan, pour the water and bring it to boil.

2 Add the shrimps and boil them over high heat for 5 minutes. After this, drain the shrimps and chill them to

room temperature.

3   Mix up together the shrimps with Splenda®, garlic
    powder, tomato sauce, and fresh parsley.

4   Add the lemon juice and stir gently.

5   Preheat the oven to 360°F.

6   Coat the slice of bread with olive oil and bake for 3
    minutes. Then place the shrimp mixture on the bread.
    The Bruschetta is cooked.

Nutrition:

Calories: 199 Fats: 3.7 Fiber: 2.1 Carbs: 15.3 Protein: 24.1
Calcium: 79 mg

Beet Feta Salad

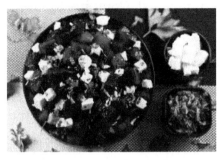

Preparation time: 15 minutes **Cooking time:** 30 minutes

Servings: 4

Ingredients:

- ✓ cups baby salad greens
- ✓ ½ sweet onion, sliced 8 small beets, trimmed
- ✓ 2 tablespoons + 1 teaspoon extra-virgin olive oil
- ✓ 1 tablespoon white wine vinegar
- ✓ 1 teaspoon Dijon mustard
- ✓ Black pepper (ground), to taste
- ✓ 2 tablespoons crumbled feta cheese
- ✓ 2 tablespoons walnut pieces

Directions:

1 Preheat an oven to 400 ⁰ F. Grease an aluminum foil with some cooking spray.

2 Add beets with 1 teaspoon of olive oil; combine and wrap foil. Bake for 30 minutes until it becomes tender. Cut beets into wedges.

3   In a mixing bowl, add remaining olive oil, vinegar, black pepper, and mustard. Combine to mix well with each other.

4   In a mixing bowl, add salad greens, onion, feta cheese, and walnuts. Combine to mix well with each other.

5   Add half of the prepared vinaigrette and toss well.

6   Add beet and combine well.

7   Drizzle remaining vinaigrette and serve fresh.

Nutrition:

Calories: 184 Fat: 9g Phosphorus: 98mg Potassium: 601mg Sodium: 235mg Carbohydrates: 19g Protein: 4g

Couscous Burgers

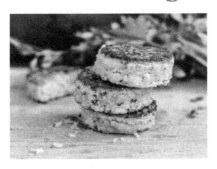

Preparation time: 25 minutes **Cooking time:** 15 minutes

Servings: 4

Ingredients:

- ✓ ½ cup chickpeas
- ✓ 2 tbsp. Chopped fresh cilantro
- ✓ Chopped fresh parsley
- ✓ 1 tbsp. Lemon juice
- ✓ 2 tsp Lemon zest
- ✓ 1 tsp Minced garlic
- ✓ 2 ½ cups Cooked couscous
- ✓ 2 Eggs, lightly beaten
- ✓ 2 tbsp. Olive oil

Directions:

1   Put the cilantro, chickpeas, parsley, lemon juice, lemon zest, and garlic in a food processor and pulse until a paste form. Transfer the chickpea mixture to a bowl, and add the eggs and couscous. Mix well.

2 Chill the mixture in the refrigerator for 1 hour.

3 Form the couscous mixture into 4 patties.

4 Heat olive oil in a skillet.

5 Place the patties in the skillet, 2 at a time, gently pressing them down with the fork of a spatula.

6 Cook for 5 minutes or until golden, and flip the patties over. Cook the other side for 5 minutes and transfer the cooked burgers to a plate covered with a paper towel.

7 Repeat with the remaining 2 burgers.

Nutrition:

Calories: 242 Total Fat: 10 g Saturated Fat: 0 g Cholesterol: 0 mg Sodium: 43 mg Total Carbs: 29 g Fiber: 0 g Sugar: 0 g Protein: 9 g

Pesto Avocado

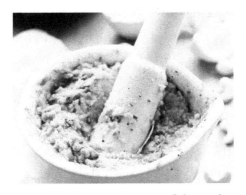

Preparation time: 15 minutes **Cooking time:** 15 minutes

Servings: 2

Ingredients:

- ✓ 1 avocado pitted, halved
- ✓ 1/3 cup Mozzarella balls, cherry size
- ✓ 1 cup fresh basil
- ✓ 1 tablespoon walnuts
- ✓ ¼ teaspoon garlic, minced
- ✓ ¾ teaspoon salt
- ✓ ¾ teaspoon ground black pepper
- ✓ tablespoons olive oil
- ✓ 1 oz. Parmesan, grated
- ✓ 1/3 cup cherry tomatoes

Directions:

1 Make pesto sauce: blend salt, minced garlic, walnuts, fresh basil, ground black pepper, and olive oil.

2   When the mixture is smooth, add grated cheese and
    pulse it for 3 seconds more.

3   Then scoop ½ flesh from the avocado halves.

4   In the mixing bowl, mix up together mozzarella balls
    and cherry tomatoes.

5   Add pesto sauce and shake it well.

6   Preheat the oven to 360F.

7   Fill the avocado halves with the cherry tomato mixture
    and bake for 10 minutes.

Nutrition:

Calories 526, Fat 53.2, Fiber 7.8, Carbs 11.7, Protein 8.2

Rutabaga Latkes

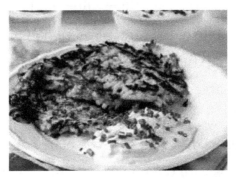

Preparation time: 15 minutes **Cooking time:** 7 minutes

Servings: 4

Ingredients:

- ✓ 1 tsp. hemp seeds
- ✓ 1 tsp. ground black pepper
- ✓ oz. rutabaga, grated
- ✓ ½ tsp. ground paprika
- ✓ tbsps. coconut flour
- ✓ 1 egg, beaten
- ✓ 1 tsp. olive oil

Directions:

1 Mix up together the hemp seeds, ground black pepper, ground paprika, and coconut flour.
2 Then add the grated rutabaga and beaten egg.
3 With the help of the fork, combine together all the ingredients into the smooth mixture.

4   Preheat the skillet for 2–3 minutes over high heat.

5   Then reduce the heat till medium and add the olive oil.

6   With the help of the fork, place the small amount of rutabaga mixture in the skillet. Flatten it gently in the shape of latkes. Cook the latkes for 3 minutes from each side.

7   After this, transfer them to the plate and repeat the same steps with the remaining rutabaga mixture.

Nutrition:

Calories: 64 Fats: 3.1 g Fiber: 3 g Carbs: 7.1 g Protein: 2.8 g

Crustless Cabbage Quiche

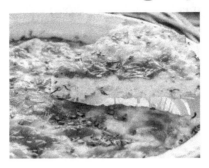

Preparation time: 10 minutes **Cooking time:** 40 minutes

Servings: 6

Ingredients:

- ✓ Olive oil cooking spray
- ✓ 2 tablespoons of extra-virgin olive oil
- ✓ 3 cups of coleslaw blend with carrots
- ✓ 3 large eggs, beaten
- ✓ 3 large egg whites, beaten
- ✓ ½ cup of half-and-half
- ✓ 1 teaspoon of dried dill weed
- ✓ ⅛ teaspoon of salt
- ✓ ⅛ teaspoon of freshly ground black pepper
- ✓ 1 cup of grated Swiss cheese

Directions:

1 Preheat the oven to 350°F. Spray pie plate (9-inch) with cooking spray and set aside.

2 In a skillet, put oil and put it in medium heat. Add the

coleslaw mix and cook for 4 to 6 minutes, stirring, until the cabbage is tender. Transfer the vegetables from the pan to a medium bowl to cool.

3   Meanwhile, in another medium bowl, combine the eggs and egg whites, half-and-half, dill, salt, and pepper, and beat to combine.

4   Stir the cabbage mixture into the egg mixture and pour into the prepared pie plate.

5   Sprinkle with the cheese.

6   Bake for 30 to 35 minutes, or until the mixture is puffed, set, and light golden brown.

Nutrition:

Calories: 203 Total Fat: 16 g Saturated Fat: 6 g Sodium: 321 mg Phosphorus: 169 mg Potassium: 155 mg Carbohydrates: 5 g Fiber: 1 g Protein: 11 g Sugar: 4 g

Vegan Chili

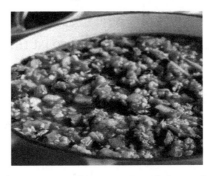

Preparation time: 10 minutes **Cooking time:** 25 minutes

Servings: 4

Ingredients:

- ✓ 1 cup cremini mushrooms, chopped
- ✓ 1 zucchini, chopped
- ✓ 1 bell pepper, diced
- ✓ 1/3 cup crushed tomatoes
- ✓ 1 oz. celery stalk, chopped
- ✓ 1 teaspoon chili powder
- ✓ 1 teaspoon salt
- ✓ ½ teaspoon chili flakes
- ✓ ½ cup of water
- ✓ 1 tablespoon olive oil
- ✓ ½ teaspoon diced garlic
- ✓ ½ teaspoon ground black pepper
- ✓ 1 teaspoon of cocoa powder
- ✓ 2 oz. Cheddar cheese, grated

Directions:

1 Pour olive oil into the pan and preheat it.

2 Add chopped mushrooms and roast them for 5 minutes. Stir them from time to time.

3 After this, add chopped zucchini and bell pepper.

4 Sprinkle the vegetables with the chili powder, salt, chili flakes, diced garlic, and ground black pepper.

5 Stir the vegetables and cook them for 5 minutes more.

6 After this, add crushed tomatoes. Mix up well.

7 Bring the mixture to boil and add water and cocoa powder. Then add celery stalk.

8 Mix up the chili well and close the lid.

9 Cook the chili for 10 minutes over medium-low heat.

10 Then transfer the cooked vegan chili to the bowls and top with the grated cheese.

Nutrition:

Nutrition: calories 123, fat 8.6, fiber 2.3, carbs 7.6, protein 5.6

Baked Eggplants Slices

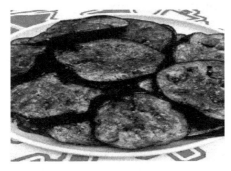

Preparation time: 15 minutes **Cooking time:** 15 minutes

Servings: 3

Ingredients:

- ✓ 1 large eggplant, finely cut
- ✓ 1 tbsp. butter, softened
- ✓ 1 tsp. minced garlic
- ✓ 1 tsp. salt

Directions:

1 Slice the eggplant season it with salt. Mix up well and leave for 10 minutes to make the vegetable 'give' bitter juice.

2 After this, dry the eggplant with a paper towel.

3 In the shallow bowl, mix up together the minced garlic and softened butter.

4 Brush every eggplant slice with the garlic mixture.

5 Line the baking tray with baking paper. Preheat the oven to 355°F.

6   Place the sliced eggplants in the tray to make 1 layer and transfer it into the oven.

7   Bake the eggplants for 15 minutes. The cooked eggplants will be tender but not soft!

Nutrition:

Calories: 81 Fats: 4.2 g Fiber: 6.5 g Carbs: 11.1 g Protein: 1.9 g

Fish and Seafood Recipes

Salmon Burgers

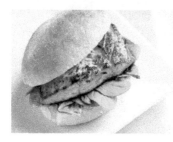

Preparation time: 10 minutes **Cooking time:** 15 minutes

Servings: 6

Ingredients:

- ✓ 16 ounces canned salmon, drained
- ✓ scallions, white and green parts, finely chopped
- ✓ ¼ cup whole-wheat bread crumbs
- ✓ 2 eggs, beaten
- ✓ 2 tablespoons chopped fresh Italian parsley leaves
- ✓ 1 tablespoon dried Italian seasoning
- ✓ Zest of 1 lemon
- ✓ 2 tablespoons extra-virgin olive oil
- ✓ ¼ cup unsweetened nonfat plain Greek yogurt
- ✓ 1 tablespoon chopped fresh dill
- ✓ 1 tablespoon capers, rinsed and chopped
- ✓ ¼ teaspoon of sea salt
- ✓ whole-wheat hamburger buns

Directions:

1   In a medium bowl, mix the salmon, scallions, bread

crumbs, eggs, parsley, Italian seasoning, and lemon zest. Form the mixture into six patties about ½-inch thick.

2   In a large nonstick skillet over medium-high heat, heat the olive oil until it shimmers.

3   Add the salmon patties. Cook for about 4 minutes per side until browned.

4   While the salmon cooks, in a small bowl, whisk the yogurt, dill, capers, and sea salt. Spread the sauce on the buns. Top with the patties and serve.

Nutrition:

Calories: 319; Protein: 28g; Total Carbohydrates: 24g; Sugars: 6g; Fiber: 3g; Total Fat: 13g; Saturated Fat: 2g; Cholesterol: 95mg; Sodium: 344mg

Shrimp Paella

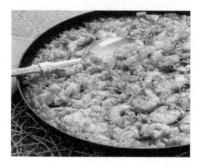

Preparation time: 5 minutes **Cooking time:** 25 minutes

Servings: 2

Ingredients:

- ✓ 1 cup cooked white rice
- ✓ 1 chopped red onion
- ✓ 1 tsp. paprika
- ✓ 1 chopped garlic clove
- ✓ 1 tbsp. olive oil
- ✓ oz. frozen cooked shrimp
- ✓ 1 chili pepper, seeded, sliced
- ✓ 1 tbsp. oregano

Directions:

1 Warm up olive oil in a large pan on medium-high heat. Add the onion and garlic and sauté for 2–3 minutes until soft. Now add the shrimp and sauté for a further 5 minutes or until heated through.

2 Now add the herbs, spices, chili, and rice with ½ cup

boiling water. Stir until everything is warm, and the water has been absorbed. Plate up and serve.

Nutrition:

Calories: 221 Protein: 17 g Carbs: 31 g Fats: 8 g Sodium: 235 mg Potassium: 176 mg Phosphorus: 189 mg

Fish Tacos

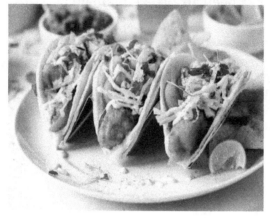

Preparation time: 10 minutes **Cooking time:** 40 minutes

Servings: 6

Ingredients:

- ✓ 1½ cup of cabbage
- ✓ ½ cup of red onion
- ✓ ½ bunch of cilantro
- ✓ 1 garlic clove
- ✓ limes
- ✓ 1 pound of cod fillets
- ✓ ½ teaspoon of ground cumin
- ✓ ½ teaspoon of chili powder
- ✓ 1 teaspoon of black pepper
- ✓ 1 tablespoon of olive oil
- ✓ ½ cup of mayonnaise
- ✓ ¼ cup of sour cream

- ✓ 2 tablespoons of milk
- ✓ (6-inch) corn tortillas

Directions:

1 Shred the cabbage, chop the onion and cilantro, and mince the garlic. Set aside.

2 Use a dish to place in the fish fillets, then squeeze half a lime juice over the fish. Sprinkle the fish fillets with the minced garlic, cumin, black pepper, chili powder, and olive oil. Turn the fish filets to coat with the marinade, then refrigerate for about 15 to 30 minutes.

3 Prepare salsa Blanca by mixing the mayonnaise, milk, sour cream, and the other half of the lime juice. Stir to combine, then place in the refrigerator to chill.

4 Broil in oven, and cover the broiler pan with aluminum foil. Broil the coated fish fillets for about 10 minutes or until the flesh becomes opaque and white and flakes easily. Remove from the oven, slightly cool, and then flake the fish into bigger pieces.

5 Heat the corn tortillas in a pan, one at a time until it becomes soft and warm, then wrap in a dish towel to keep them warm.

6 To assemble the tacos, place a piece of the fish on the tortilla, topping with the salsa blanca, cabbage, cilantro, red onion, and the lime wedges.

Nutrition:

Calories: 363 Protein: 18g Carbohydrat:es 30g Fat: 19g
Cholesterol: 40mg Sodium: 194mg Potassium: 507mg
Phosphorus: 327mg Fiber: 4.3g

Pan-Roasted Salmon with Gremolata

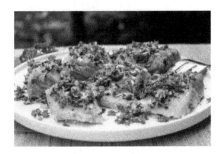

Preparation time: 15 minutes **Cooking time:** 10 minutes

Servings: 6

Ingredients:

- ✓ 1½ pounds skin-on salmon fillet, cut into four pieces
- ✓ 1 teaspoon sea salt, divided
- ✓ ¼ teaspoon freshly ground black pepper
- ✓ tablespoons extra-virgin olive oil
- ✓ 1 bunch fresh Italian parsley leaves, finely chopped
- ✓ 1 garlic clove, minced
- ✓ Zest of 1 lemon, finely grated (see tip)

Directions:

1 Preheat the oven to 350°F.
2 Season the salmon with ½ teaspoon of salt and pepper.
3 In a large, ovenproof skillet over medium-high heat, heat the olive oil until it shimmers.
4 Add the salmon to the skillet, skin-side down. Cook for

about 5 minutes, gently pressing on the salmon with a spatula, until the skin crisps. Transfer the pan to the oven and cook the salmon for 3 to 4 minutes more until opaque.

5   In a small bowl, stir together the parsley, garlic, lemon zest, and remaining ½ teaspoon of sea salt. Sprinkle the mixture over the salmon and serve.

Nutrition:

Calories: 214; Protein: 22g; Total Carbohydrates: <1g; Sugars: <1g; Fiber: <1g; Total Fat: 14g; Saturated Fat: 2g; Cholesterol: 50mg; Sodium: 522mg

Baked Fennel & Garlic Sea Bass

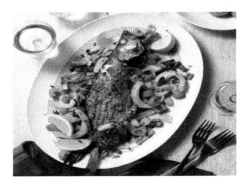

Preparation time: 5 minutes **Cooking time:** 15 minutes

Servings: 2

Ingredients:

- ✓ 1 lemon
- ✓ ½ sliced fennel bulb
- ✓ oz. sea bass fillets
- ✓ 1 tsp. black pepper
- ✓ garlic cloves

Directions:

1   Preheat the oven to 375°F. Sprinkle the black pepper over the fillets. Slice the fennel bulb and garlic cloves. Add 1 salmon fillet and half the fennel and garlic to one sheet of baking paper or tin foil.

2   Squeeze in ½ lemon juices. Repeat for the other fillet. Fold and add to the oven for 12–15 minutes or until the fish is thoroughly cooked through.

3   Meanwhile, add the boiling water to your couscous, cover, and allow to steam.

Nutrition:

Calories: 221 Protein: 14 g Carbs: 3 g Fats: 2 g Sodium: 119 mg Potassium: 398 mg Phosphorus: 149 mg

Asparagus Shrimp Linguini

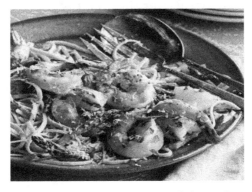

Preparation time: 10 minutes **Cooking time:** 5 minutes

Servings: 2

Ingredients:

- ✓ ounces of uncooked linguini
- ✓ 1 tablespoon of olive oil
- ✓ 1¾ cups of asparagus
- ✓ ½ cup of unsalted butter
- ✓ garlic cloves
- ✓ ounces of cream cheese
- ✓ 2 tablespoons of fresh parsley
- ✓ ¾ teaspoon of dried basil
- ✓ ⅔ cup of dry white wine
- ✓ ½ pound of peeled and cooked shrimp

Directions:

1 Preheat oven to 350° F. Cook the linguini in boiling water until it becomes tender, then drain.

2   Place the asparagus on a baking sheet, then spread two tablespoons of oil over the asparagus. Bake for about 7 to 8 minutes or until it is tender.

3   Remove baked asparagus from the oven and place it on a plate. Cut the asparagus into pieces of medium-sized once cooled.

4   Mince the garlic and chop the parsley.

5   Melt ½ cup of butter in a large skillet with the minced garlic. Stir in the cream cheese, mixing as it melts.

6   Stir in the parsley and basil, then simmer for about 5 minutes. Mix either in boiling water or dry white wine, stirring until the sauce becomes smooth.

7   Add the cooked shrimp and asparagus, then stir and heat until it is evenly warm.

Nutrition:

Calories: 544 Protein: 21g Carbohydrates: 43g Fat: 32g
Cholesterol: 188mg Sodium: 170mg Potassium: 402mg
Phosphorus: 225mg Fiber: 2.4g

Fish Kebab

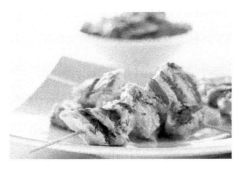

Preparation time: 20 minutes **Cooking time:** 20 minutes

Servings: 6

Ingredients:

- ✓ tablespoons extra-virgin olive oil, plus more for the grill
- ✓ Juice of 2 oranges
- ✓ 1 tablespoon Dijon mustard
- ✓ 1 teaspoons dried tarragon
- ✓ 1-half tsp. sea salt
- ✓ 1-third tsp. freshly ground black pepper
- ✓ pounds swordfish, cut into 1½-inch pieces
- ✓ 2 red bell peppers, cut into pieces

Directions:

1   In a medium bowl, whisk the olive oil, orange juice, mustard, tarragon, sea salt, and pepper.

2   Add the swordfish and toss to coat. Let sit for 10 minutes. Heat a grill or grill pan to medium-high heat and brush it with oil.

3   Thread the swordfish and red bell peppers onto six
     wooden skewers (see tip). Cook for 6 to 8 minutes,
     turning until the fish is opaque.

Nutrition:

Calories: 326; Protein: 33g; Total Carbohydrates: 11g; Sugars: 8g; Fiber: 2g; Total Fat: 18g; Saturated Fat: 1g; Cholesterol: 0mg; Sodium: 187mg

Cod & Green Bean Risotto

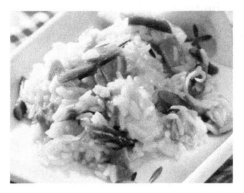

Preparation time: 5 minutes **Cooking time:** 40 minutes

Servings: 2

Ingredients:

- ✓ ½ cup arugula
- ✓ 1 finely diced white onion
- ✓ oz. cod fillet
- ✓ 1 cup white rice
- ✓ lemon wedges
- ✓ 1 cup boiling water
- ✓ ¼ tsp. black pepper
- ✓ 1 cup low-sodium chicken broth
- ✓ 1 tbsp. extra-virgin olive oil
- ✓ ½ cup green beans

Directions:

1 Warm up oil in a large pan over medium heat. Sauté the chopped onion for 5 minutes until soft and before

adding in the rice and stirring for 1–2 minutes.

2   Combine the broth with the boiling water. Add half of the liquid to the pan and stir. Slowly add the rest of the liquid while continuously stirring for up to 20–30 minutes.

3   Stir in the green beans to the risotto. Place the fish on top of the rice, cover, and steam for 10 minutes.

4   Use your fork to break up the fish fillets and stir into the rice. Sprinkle with freshly ground pepper to serve and a squeeze of fresh lemon. Serve with lemon wedges and arugula.

Nutrition:

Calories: 221 Protein: 12 g Carbs: 29 g

Oven-Fried Southern Style Catfish

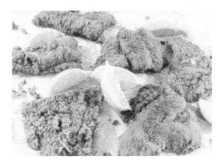

Preparation time: 10 minutes **Cooking time:** 35 minutes

Servings: 4

Ingredients:

- ✓ 1 egg white
- ✓ ½ cup of all-purpose flour
- ✓ ¼ cup of cornmeal
- ✓ ¼ cup of panko bread crumbs
- ✓ 1 teaspoon of salt-free Cajun seasoning
- ✓ 1 pound of catfish fillets

Directions:

1 Heat oven to 450° F. Use cooking spray to spray a non-stick baking sheet.

2 Using a bowl, beat the egg white until very soft peaks are formed. Don't over-beat.

3 Use a sheet of wax paper and place the flour over it.

4 Using a different sheet of wax paper to combine and mix the cornmeal, panko and the Cajun seasoning.

5   Cut the catfish fillet into four pieces, then dip the fish in the flour, shaking off the excess.

6   Dip coated fish in the egg white, rolling into the cornmeal mixture.

7   Place the fish on the baking pan. Repeat with the remaining fish fillets.

8   Use cooking spray to spray over the fish fillets. Bake for about 10 to 12 minutes or until the sides of the fillets become browned and crisp.

Nutrition:

Calories 250 Protein 22g Carbohydrates 19g Fat 10g Cholesterol 53mg Sodium 124mg Potassium 401mg Phosphorus 262mg Fiber 1.2g

Sardine Fish Cakes

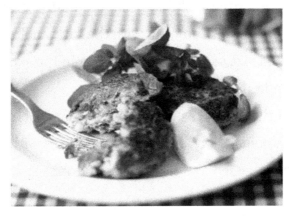

Preparation time: 15 minutes **Cooking time:** 15 minutes

Servings: 4

Ingredients:

- ✓ oz. sardines, canned, drained
- ✓ 1/3 cup shallot, chopped
- ✓ 1 tsp. chili flakes
- ✓ ½ tsp. salt
- ✓ tbsps. wheat flour, whole grain
- ✓ 1 egg, beaten
- ✓ 1 tbsp. chives, chopped
- ✓ 1 tsp. olive oil
- ✓ 1 tsp. butter

Directions:

1　Put the butter in your skillet and dissolve it. Add the shallot and cook it until translucent. After this, transfer the shallot to the mixing bowl.

2 Add the sardines, chili flakes, salt, flour, egg, chives, and mix up until smooth with the fork's help. Make the medium size cakes and place them in the skillet, and then add the olive oil.

3 Roast the fish cakes for 3 minutes from each side over medium heat. Dry the cooked fish cakes with a paper towel if needed and transfer them to the serving plates.

Nutrition:

Calories: 221 Fats: 12.2 g Fiber: 0.1 g Carbs: 5.4 g Protein: 21.3 g Phosphorus: 188.7 mg Potassium: 160.3 mg Sodium: 452.6 mg

Shrimp Quesadilla

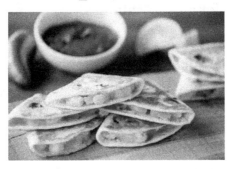

Preparation time: 15 minutes **Cooking time:** 15 minutes

Servings: 4

Ingredients:

- ✓ ounces of raw shrimp
- ✓ tablespoons of cilantro
- ✓ 1 tablespoon of lemon juice
- ✓ ¼ teaspoon of ground cumin
- ✓ ⅛ teaspoon of cayenne pepper
- ✓ flour burrito-sized tortillas
- ✓ 2 tablespoons of sour cream
- ✓ teaspoons of salsa
- ✓ 2 tablespoons of shredded jalapeno cheddar cheese

Directions:

1 Peel the shrimp, rinse, and then cut into pieces of bite-size. Dice the cilantro.

2 Use a zip-lock bag to combine and mix the cilantro, lemon juice, cumin, and cayenne pepper to make the

marinade. Add the pieces of shrimp and put aside to marinate for about 5 minutes.

3   Heat a skillet over medium heat and add the shrimp with the marinade. Stir-fry for about 1 to 2 minutes or until the shrimp is orange in color. Remove the skillet from heat and spoon out the shrimp, leaving marinade.

4   Add the sour cream to the skillet with the leftover marinade. Stir to mix.

5   Use a large skillet or microwave to heat the tortillas, then spread two teaspoons of salsa over each tortilla. Top with ½ of the shrimp mixture, sprinkling with one tablespoon of cheddar cheese.

6   Spoon out one tablespoon of the sour cream mixture from step 4 on top of the shrimp, fold the tortilla into half, turning over in skillet to heat, then remove from the pan. Repeat the same process with the second tortilla and with the remaining shrimp, cheese and marinade Cut each of the tortillas into four pieces, and serve.

Nutrition:

Calories 318 Protein 20g Carbohydrates 26g Fat 15g Cholesterol 118mg Sodium 398mg Potassium 276mg Phosphorus 243mg Fiber 1.2g

Spanish Cod in Sauce

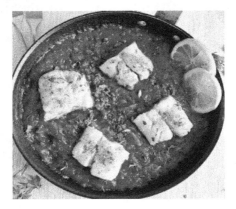

Preparation time: 15 minutes **Cooking time:** 15 minutes

Servings: 4

Ingredients:

- ✓ 1 tsp. tomato paste
- ✓ 1 tsp. garlic, diced
- ✓ 1 white onion, sliced
- ✓ 1 jalapeño pepper, chopped
- ✓ 1/3 cup chicken stock
- ✓ oz. Spanish cod fillet
- ✓ 1 tsp. paprika
- ✓ 1 tsp. salt

Directions:

1   Pour the chicken stock into the saucepan.

2   Add the tomato paste and mix up the liquid until homogenous. Add the garlic, onion, jalapeño pepper,

117

paprika, and salt.

3 Bring the liquid to boil and then simmer it. Chop the cod fillet and add it to the tomato liquid.

4 Simmer the fish for 10 minutes over low heat. Serve the fish in the bowls with tomato sauce.

Nutrition:

Calories: 113 Fats: 1.2 g Fiber: 1.9 g Carbs: 7.2 g Protein: 18.9 g Potassium: 659 mg Sodium: 597 mg Phosphorus: 18 mg

Creamy Crab over Salmon

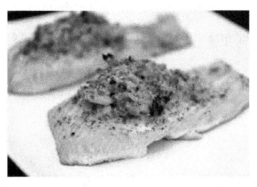

Preparation time: 15 minutes **Cooking time:** 15 minutes

Servings: 4

Ingredients:

- ✓ ¼ cup olive oil, divided
- ✓ 2 (4 ounce) fillets salmon
- ✓ 1 teaspoon dried oregano
- ✓ 1 pinch ground white pepper
- ✓ 1 3/4 cups soy milk
- ✓ ounces' fresh crabmeat
- ✓ 1 teaspoon lemon juice

Directions:

1 Heat a small amount of olive oil in a non-stick skillet over medium heat. Season salmon with oregano and white pepper; cook in skillet until the flesh flakes easily with a fork, 7 to 10 minutes per side.

2 While fish cooks, whisk the remaining olive oil and the

soy milk together in a saucepan over medium-low heat; cook, stirring regularly, until it thickens, 3 to 5 minutes. Remove the saucepan from heat and stir crab meat into the sauce.

3 Transfer cooked cod to plates and spoon sauce over the fish.

Nutrition:

Calories: 258 Total Fat: 16.5 g Saturated Fat: 2.5 g Cholesterol: 40 mg Sodium: 395 mg Total Carbohydrates: 11.4 g Dietary Fiber: 1 g Total Sugar 6.1 g Protein: 17.3 g Calcium: 37 mg Iron: 1 mg Potassium: 160 mg Potassium: 120 mg

Marinated Salmon Steak

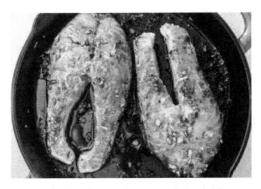

Preparation time: 10 minutes **Cooking time:** 15 minutes

Servings: 4

Ingredients:

- ✓ ¼ cup lime juice
- ✓ ¼ cup soy sauce
- ✓ tbsps. olive oil
- ✓ 1 tbsp. lemon juice
- ✓ tbsps. chopped fresh parsley
- ✓ ½ tsp. chopped fresh oregano
- ✓ ½ tsp. ground black pepper
- ✓ (4 oz.) salmon steaks

Directions:

1   In a large non-reactive dish, mix together the lime juice, soy sauce, olive oil, lemon juice, parsley, garlic, oregano, and pepper. Place the salmon steaks in the marinade and turn to coat. Cover, and refrigerate for at

least 30 minutes.

2   Preheat the grill for high heat.

3   Lightly oil the grill grate. Cook the salmon steaks for 5–6 minutes, then baste with the marinade. Cook for an additional 5 minutes, or to the desired doneness. Discard any remaining marinade.

Nutrition:

Calories: 108 Fats: 8.4 g Saturated Fats: 1.2 g
Cholesterol: 9 mg Sodium: 910 mg Carbs: 3.6 g
Fiber: 0.4 g Sugars: 1.7 g

Fish Chili with Lentils

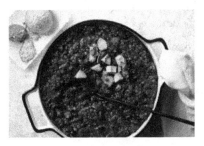

Preparation time: 10 minutes **Cooking time:** 40 minutes

Servings: 4

Ingredients:

- ✓ 1 red pepper, chopped
- ✓ 1 yellow onion, diced
- ✓ 1 tsp. ground black pepper
- ✓ 1 tsp. butter
- ✓ 1 jalapeño pepper, chopped
- ✓ ½ cup lentils
- ✓ 3 cups chicken stock
- ✓ 1 tsp. salt
- ✓ 1 tbsp. tomato paste
- ✓ 1 tsp. chili pepper
- ✓ tbsps. fresh cilantro, chopped
- ✓ 8 oz. cod, chopped

Directions:

1   Place the butter, red pepper, onion, and ground black pepper in the saucepan. Roast the vegetables for 5

minutes over medium heat.

2 Then add the chopped jalapeño pepper, lentils, and chili pepper. Mix up the mixture well and add the chicken stock and tomato paste. Stir until homogenous.

3 Add the cod. Close the lid and cook the chili for 20 minutes over medium heat.

Nutrition:

Calories: 187 Fats: 2.3 g Carbs: 21.3 g Protein: 20.6 g Phosphorus: 50 mg Potassium: 281 mg Sodium: 43.8 mg

Meat Recipes

Ground Lamb with Harissa

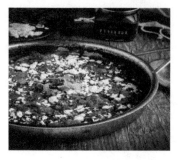

Preparation time: 15 minutes **Cooking time:** 1hr 20 minutes

Servings: 4

Ingredients:

- ✓ 1 tbsp. extra-virgin olive oil
- ✓ red peppers, seeded and chopped finely
- ✓ 1 yellow onion, chopped finely
- ✓ garlic cloves, chopped finely
- ✓ 1 tsp. ground cumin
- ✓ ½ tsp. ground turmeric
- ✓ ¼ tsp. ground cinnamon
- ✓ ¼ tsp. ground ginger 1
- ✓ ½ lb. lean ground lamb
- ✓ Salt to taste
- ✓ 1 (¼ –½-oz.) can diced red bell peppers
- ✓ 2 tbsps. Harissa
- ✓ 1 cup water
- ✓ Chopped fresh cilantro, for garnishing

Directions:

1   In a large pan, heat the oil over medium-high heat.

2   Add the bell pepper, onion, and garlic and sauté for around 5 minutes.

3   Add the spices and sauté for around 1 minute.

4   Add the lamb and salt and cook for approximately 5 minutes, getting into pieces.

5   Stir in the red bell peppers, harissa, and water and provide with a boil.

6   Reduce the warmth to low and simmer, covered for about 1 hour.

7   Serve hot with the harissa.

Nutrition:

Calories: 441 Fats: 12 g Carbs: 24 g Fiber: 10 g Protein: 36 g

Roast Beef

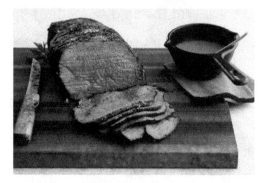

Preparation time: 25 minutes **Cooking time:** 55 minutes

Servings: 3

Ingredients:

✓ Quality rump or sirloin tip roast.

Directions:

1 Place in roasting pan on a shallow rack

2 Season with pepper and herbs.

3 Insert meat thermometer in the center or thickest part of the roast.

4 Roast to the desired degree of doneness.

5 After removing from over for about 15 minutes, let it chill.

6 In the end, the roast should be moist.

Nutrition:

Calories: 158 Protein: 24g Fat: 6g Carbs: 0g Phosphorus: 206mg Potassium: 328mg Sodium: 55mg.

Open-Faced Beef Stir-Up

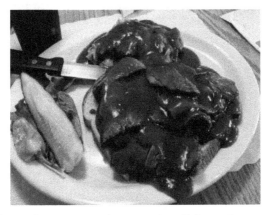

Preparation time: 10 minutes **Cooking time:** 10 minutes

Servings: 6

Ingredients:

- ✓ ½ pound 95% lean ground beef
- ✓ ½ cup chopped sweet onion
- ✓ ½ cup shredded cabbage
- ✓ ¼ cup herb pesto
- ✓ hamburger buns, bottom halves only

Directions:

1 Sauté the beef and onion for 6 minutes or until the beef is cooked.

2 Add the cabbage and sauté for 3 minutes more.

3 Stir in pesto and heat for 1 minute.

4 Divide the beef mixture into 6 portions and serve each on the bottom half of a hamburger bun, open-face.

Nutrition:

Calories: 120 Fat: 3 g Phosphorus: 106 mg Potassium: 198 mg Sodium: 134 mg Protein: 11 g

Grilled Lamb Chops

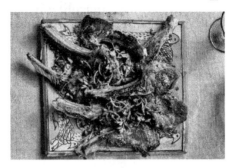

Preparation time: 10 minutes **Cooking time:** 10 minutes

Servings: 4

Ingredients:

- ✓ 1 tbsp. fresh ginger, grated
- ✓ 4 garlic cloves, chopped roughly
- ✓ 1 tsp. ground cumin
- ✓ ½ tsp. red chili powder
- ✓ Salt and freshly ground black pepper, to taste
- ✓ 1 tbsp. essential olive oil
- ✓ 1 tbsp. fresh lemon juice
- ✓ lamb chops, finely cut

Directions:

1. In a bowl, mix together all the ingredients except the chops. With a hand blender, blend till a smooth mixture forms.
2. Add chops and coat generously with the mixture.
3. Refrigerate to marinate overnight.

4   Preheat the barbecue grill till hot. Grease the grill grate.

5   Grill the chops for approximately 3 minutes per side.

Nutrition:

Calories: 227 Fats: 12 g Carbs: 1 g Protein: 30 g

Country Fried Steak

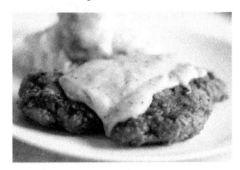

Preparation time: 10 minutes **Cooking time:** 1 hr 20 minutes

Servings: 3

Ingredients:

- ✓ One large onion
- ✓ ½ cup flour
- ✓ tbsps. Vegetable oil
- ✓ ¼ tsp. pepper
- ✓ 1½ lbs. round steak
- ✓ ½ tsp. Paprika.

Directions:

1. Trim excess fat from steak.
2. Cut into small pieces.
3. Combine flour, paprika, and pepper and mix.
4. Preheat skillet with oil.
5. Cook steak on both sides.
6. Add water (150 ml) and stir around the skillet.

Nutrition:

Calories: 248 Protein: 30g Fat: 10g Carbs: 5g Phosphorus: 190mg Potassium: 338mg Sodium: 60mg.

Pork with Bell Pepper

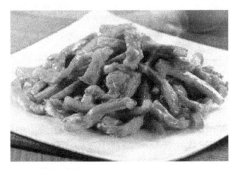

Preparation time: 15 minutes **Cooking time:** 15 minutes

Servings: 1

Ingredients:

- ✓ 1 tablespoon fresh ginger, chopped finely
- ✓ 4 garlic cloves, chopped finely
- ✓ 1 cup fresh cilantro, chopped and divided
- ✓ ¼ cup plus
- ✓ 1 tablespoon olive oil, divided
- ✓ 1-pound tender pork, trimmed, sliced thinly
- ✓ 2 onions, sliced thinly
- ✓ 1 green bell pepper, seeded and sliced thinly
- ✓ 1 tablespoon fresh lime juice

Directions:

1 In a substantial bowl, mix ginger, garlic, ½ cup of cilantro, and ¼ cup of oil.

2 Add pork and coat with mixture generously.

3 Refrigerate to marinate for a couple of hours.

4   Heat a big skillet on medium-high heat.

5   Add pork mixture and stir fry for approximately 4-5 minutes. Transfer the pork right into a bowl.

6   In the same skillet, heat the remaining oil on medium heat. Add onion and sauté for approximately 3 minutes.

7   Stir in bell pepper and stir fry for about 3 minutes.

8   Stir in pork, lime juice, and remaining cilantro and cook for about 2 minutes.

9   Serve hot.

Nutrition:

Calories: 429 Fat: 19 g Phosphorus: 36 mg Potassium: 57 mg Sodium: 31 mg Carbohydrates: 26 g Fiber: 9 g Protein: 35 g.

Beef Ragu

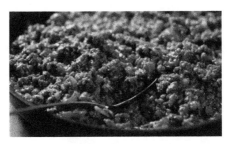

Preparation time: 10 minutes **Cooking time:** 20 minutes

Servings: 2

Ingredients:

- ✓ ¼ cup packaged pesto
- ✓ 1 tsp. salt 2 large zucchinis, cut into noodle strips
- ✓ 1 tbsp. olive oil
- ✓ ¼ lb. ground beef
- ✓ tbsp. fresh parsley, chopped

Directions:

1. Heat the oil in a skillet over medium heat and cook the ground beef until thoroughly cooked, around 5 minutes. Discard excess fat.
2. Add the packaged pesto sauce and season with salt.
3. Then add the chopped parsley and cook for 3 more minutes. Set aside.
4. In the same saucepan, place the zucchini noodles and cook for 5 minutes. Turn off the heat and then add the cooked meat. Mix well.

5   Serve and enjoy.

Nutrition:

Calories: 353 Fats: 30 g Saturated Fat: 6 g Carbs: 2 g Net Carbs: 1.3 g Protein: 19 g Sugar: 0.3 g Fiber: 0.7 g Sodium: 1481 mg Potassium: 341 mg

Beef Keagan

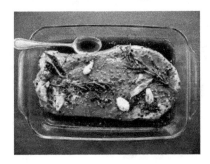

Preparation time: 10 minutes **Cooking time:** 20 minutes

Servings: 2

Ingredients:

- ✓ 1 1/2 cups lemon juice
- ✓ tablespoons Worcestershire sauce
- ✓ Black pepper to taste
- ✓ 1 bunch of green onions
- ✓ 1 pound beef flank steak.

Directions:

1. Pour lemon juice, Worcestershire sauce, and black pepper in a large, glass bowl.
2. Cover the bowl with plastic wrap and place it at room temperature for one hour until the meat turns a grayish-brown color and appears cooked.

Nutrition:

Calories: 161 Total Fat: 5.2g Sodium: 118mg Protein: 23.5g Potassium: 392mg Phosphorus: 225mg.

Ground Pork with Water Chestnuts

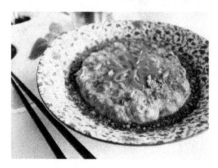

Preparation time: 15 minutes **Cooking time:** 20 minutes

Servings: 1

Ingredients:

- ✓ 1 tablespoon plus
- ✓ 1 teaspoon coconut oil
- ✓ 1 tablespoon fresh ginger, minced
- ✓ 1 bunch scallion (white and green parts separated), chopped
- ✓ 1-pound lean ground pork
- ✓ Salt, to taste
- ✓ 1 tablespoon 5-spice powder
- ✓ 1 (18-ounce) can water chestnuts, drained and chopped
- ✓ 1 tablespoon organic honey
- ✓ tablespoons fresh lime juice

Directions:

1 In a big heavy-bottomed skillet, heat oil on high heat.
2 Add ginger and scallion whites and sauté for

approximately ½-1½ minutes.

3   Add pork and cook for approximately 4-5 minutes.

4   Drain the extra fat from the skillet.

5   Add salt and 5-spice powder and cook for approximately 2-3 minutes

6   Add scallion greens and remaining ingredients and cook, stirring continuously for about 1-2 minutes.

Nutrition:

Calories: 520 Fat: 30 g Phosphorus: 20 mg Potassium: 120 mg Sodium: 9 mg Carbohydrates: 37 g Fiber: 4 g Protein: 25 g.

Mouthwatering Beef and Chili Stew

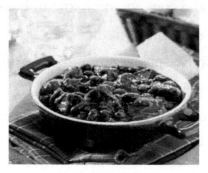

Preparation time: 15 minutes **Cooking time:** 7 hr

Servings: 6

Ingredients:

- ✓ 1/2 medium red onion
- ✓ 1 tablespoon vegetable oil
- ✓ 10 ounce of flat-cut beef brisket, whole
- ✓ ½ cup low sodium stock
- ✓ ¾ cup of water
- ✓ ½ tablespoon honey
- ✓ ½ tablespoon chili powder
- ✓ ½ teaspoon smoked paprika
- ✓ ½ teaspoon dried thyme
- ✓ 1 teaspoon black pepper
- ✓ 1 tablespoon corn starch

Directions:

1   Throw the sliced onion into the slow cooker first.

2   Add a splash of oil to a large hot skillet and briefly seal

the beef.

3   Remove the beef from the skillet and place it in the slow cooker.

4   Add the stock, water, honey, and spices to the same skillet you cooked the beef.

5   Loosen the browned bits from the bottom of the pan with a spatula. (Hint: These brown bits at the bottom are called "the fond.")

6   Allow the juice to simmer until the volume is reduced by about half.

7   Pour the juice over beef in the slow cooker.

8   Set slow cooker on low and cook for approximately 7 hours. Take the beef out of the slow cooker and onto a platter.

9   to a simmer. water. thickened.

10 Shred-it with two forks.

11 Pour the remaining juice into a saucepan. Bring it.

12 Add to the juice and cook until slightly. For a thicker sauce, simmer and reduce the juice a bit more before adding cornstarch.

13 Serve with sauce

Nutrition:

Calories: 128 Protein: 13g Carbohydrates: 6g Fat: 6g

Cholesterol: 39mg Sodium: 228mg Potassium: 202mg

Phosphorus: 119mg Calcium: 16mg Fiber: 1g.

Beef Brochettes

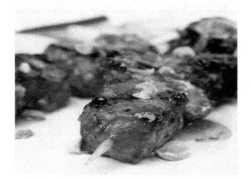

Preparation time: 15 minutes **Cooking time:** 1 hr

Servings: 1

Ingredients:

- ✓ 1 ½ cups pineapple chunks
- ✓ 1 large onion, sliced
- ✓ 2 lbs. thick steak
- ✓ 1 bell pepper, medium, sliced
- ✓ 1 bay leaf
- ✓ ¼ cup vegetable oil
- ✓ ½ cup lemon juice
- ✓ 2 crushed garlic cloves

Directions:

1. Cut the beef into cubes and put them in a plastic bag.
2. Place the other ingredients in a small bowl.
3. Mix the ingredients and pour the mix over the beef cubes.

4   Seal the bag and refrigerate for 3 to 5 hours.

5   Grill about 9 minutes on each side.

Nutrition:

Calories: 304 Protein: 35 g Fats: 15 g Carbs: 11 g Phosphorus: 264 mg Potassium: 388 mg Sodium: 70 mg

Chicken with Mushrooms

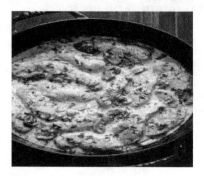

Preparation time: 15 minutes **Cooking time:** 45 minutes

Servings: 2

Ingredients:

- ✓ 2 tablespoons light sour cream
- ✓ ¼ cup all-purpose flour
- ✓ 1 cup no salt added chicken broth
- ✓ 1 tablespoon Dijon mustard
- ✓ ¼ teaspoon dried thyme
- ✓ 4 chicken breasts
- ✓ 1½ cups mushrooms, quartered
- ✓ 1 tablespoon non-hydrogenated margarine
- ✓ Fresh ground pepper and chopped fresh parsley, to taste
- ✓ 3 chopped green onions

Directions:

1 Mix 2 tablespoon of chicken broth, mustard, sour cream, and 2 teaspoon flour. Set aside.

2   Sprinkle chicken with pepper and thyme. Dredge in flour. Melt margarine on medium-low heat in a large non-stick pan. Cook chicken for 15-20 minutes per side. Remove from heat and keep warm.

3   Add mushrooms to another pan.

4   Add sour cream mixture and green onions and cook until thickened.

5   Pour over chicken. Garnish with parsley and pepper.

Nutrition:

Protein: 25.4 g Phosphorus: 29 mg Potassium: 142 mg Sodium: 17 mg Carbohydrates: 5 g Fat: 4 g Calories: 161.

Beef and Three Pepper Stew

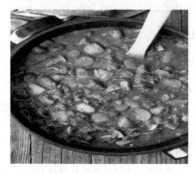

Preparation time: 15 minutes **Cooking time:** 6 hr

Servings: 6

Ingredients:

- ✓ 10 ounce of flat-cut beef brisket, whole
- ✓ 1 teaspoon of dried thyme
- ✓ 1 teaspoon of black pepper
- ✓ 1 clove garlic
- ✓ ½ cup of green onion, thinly sliced
- ✓ ½ cup of low sodium chicken stock
- ✓ cups of water
- ✓ 1 large green bell pepper, sliced
- ✓ 1 large red bell pepper, sliced
- ✓ 1 large yellow bell pepper, sliced
- ✓ 1 large red onion, sliced.

Directions:

1 Combine the beef, thyme, pepper, garlic, green onion, stock, and water in a slow cooker.

2   Leave it all to cook on High for 4-5 hours until tender. Remove the beef from the slow cooker and let it cool.

3   Shred the beef with two forks and remove any excess fat.

4   Place the shredded beef back into the slow cooker.

5   Add the sliced peppers and the onion.

6   Cook this on high heat for 40-60 minutes until the vegetables are tender.

Nutrition:

Protein: 14g Carbohydrates: 9g Fat: 5g Cholesterol: 39mg Sodium: 179mg Potassium: 390mg Phosphorus: 141mg Calcium: 33mg Fiber: 2g.

Pork Souvlaki

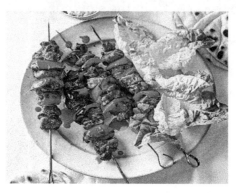

Preparation time: 20 minutes **Cooking time:** 12 minutes

Servings: 8

Ingredients:

- ✓ 3 tbsps. olive oil
- ✓ 2 tbsps. lemon juice
- ✓ 1 tsp. garlic, minced
- ✓ 1 tbsp. fresh oregano, chopped
- ✓ ¼ tsp. ground black pepper
- ✓ 1 lb. pork leg, cut into 2-inch cubes

Directions:

1 In a bowl, stir together the lemon juice, olive oil, garlic, oregano, and pepper.

2 Add the pork cubes and toss to coat.

3 Cover and place the bowl in the refrigerator for 2 hours to marinate.

4 Thread the pork chunks onto 8 wooden skewers that

have been soaked in water.

5   Preheat the barbecue to medium-high heat.

6   Grill the pork skewers for about 12 minutes, turning
    once, until just cooked through but still juicy.

Nutrition:

Calories: 95 Fats: 4 g Phosphorus: 125 mg Potassium: 230 mg
Sodium: 29 mg Protein: 13 g

Chicken Meatballs Curry

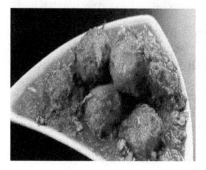

Preparation time: 20 minutes **Cooking time:** 25 minutes

Servings: 4

Ingredients:

- ✓ 1 lb. lean ground chicken
- ✓ 1 tbsp. onion paste
- ✓ 1 tsp. fresh ginger paste
- ✓ 1 tsp. garlic paste
- ✓ 1 green chili, chopped finely
- ✓ 1 tbsp. fresh cilantro leaves, chopped
- ✓ 1 tsp. ground coriander
- ✓ ½ tsp. cumin seeds
- ✓ ½ tsp. red chili powder
- ✓ ½ tsp. ground turmeric
- ✓ Salt to taste

For the Curry:

- ✓ tbsps. extra-virgin olive oil
- ✓ ½ tsp. cumin seeds

- ✓ 1 (1-inch) cinnamon stick
- ✓ whole cloves
- ✓ whole green cardamoms
- ✓ 1 whole black cardamom
- ✓ onions, chopped
- ✓ 1 tsp. fresh ginger, minced
- ✓ 1 tsp. garlic, minced
- ✓ whole red bell peppers, chopped finely
- ✓ tsp. ground coriander
- ✓ 1 tsp. garam masala powder
- ✓ ½ tsp. ground nutmeg
- ✓ ½ tsp. red chili powder
- ✓ ½ tsp. ground turmeric
- ✓ Salt to taste
- ✓ 1 cup water
- ✓ Chopped fresh cilantro for garnishing

Directions:

1 To make the meatballs, add all the ingredients into a bowl and mix till well combined.

2 Warm up the oil over medium heat in a big, deep skillet. Add the meatballs and fry for approximately 3–5 minutes or till browned from all sides. Transfer the meatballs to a bowl.

3 In the same skillet, add the cumin seeds, cinnamon

stick, cloves, green cardamom, and black cardamom and sauté for approximately 1 minute.

4 Add the onions and sauté for around 4–5 minutes, then put the ginger and garlic paste and sauté for 1 minute. Add the tomato and spices and cook, crushing with the back of the spoon for about 2–3 minutes.

5 Add the water and meatballs and bring to a boil. Reduce the heat to low. Simmer for approximately 10 minutes. Serve hot with cilantro.

Nutrition:

Calories: 421 Fats: 8 g Carbs: 18 g Fiber: 5 g Protein: 34 g

Snack & Sandwiches

Chicken Lettuce Wraps

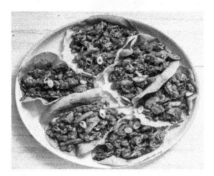

Preparation time: 30 minutes **Cooking time:** 0 minutes

Servings: 8

Ingredients:

- ✓ 6 ounces, minced Cooked chicken breast
- ✓ Scallion
- ✓ 1 Red apple
- ✓ ½ cup Bean sprouts
- ✓ ¼ English cucumber
- ✓ 1 Juice of lime
- ✓ 1 Zest of lime
- ✓ 2 tbsp. Chopped fresh cilantro
- ✓ ½ tsp Chinese spice powder
- ✓ 8 Boston lettuce leaves

Directions:

1 In a bowl, mix the scallions, chicken, apple, cucumber, bean sprouts, lime juice, lime zest, cilantro, and five-spice powder. Spoon the chicken mixture evenly among

the eight lettuce leaves.

2 Wrap the lettuce around the chicken mixture and serve.

Nutrition:

Calories: 51 Fat: 2g Carb: 2g Phosphorus: 56mg Potassium: 110mg Sodium: 16mg Protein: 7g

Eggplant Sandwich

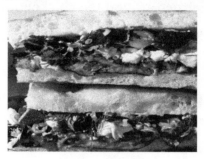

Preparation time: 30 minutes **Cooking time:** 30 minutes

Servings: 2

Ingredients:

- ✓ 1 eggplant, sliced
- ✓ 2 teaspoons parsley, dried
- ✓ Salt and black pepper to the taste
- ✓ ½ cup vegan breadcrumbs
- ✓ ½ teaspoon Italian seasoning
- ✓ ½ teaspoon garlic powder
- ✓ ½ teaspoon onion powder
- ✓ ½ tablespoons almond milk
- ✓ 4 vegan bread slices
- ✓ Cooking spray
- ✓ ¾ cup tomato sauce
- ✓ A handful basil, chopped

Directions:

1 Season eggplant slices with salt and pepper, leave aside

for 30 minutes and then pat dry them well.

2 In a bowl, mix parsley with breadcrumbs, Italian seasoning, onion and garlic powder, salt and black pepper and stir.

3 In another bowl, mix milk with vegan mayo and also stir well. Brush eggplant slices with mayo mix, dip them in breadcrumbs mix, place them on a lined baking sheet, spray with cooking oil, introduce baking sheet in your air fryer's basket and cook them at 400 degrees F for 15 minutes, flipping them halfway.

4 Brush each bread slice with olive oil and arrange 2 of them on a working surface.

5 Add baked eggplant slices, spread tomato sauce and basil and top with the other bread slices, greased side down.

6 Divide between plates and serve.

Nutrition:

Calories 324, Fat 16, Fiber 4, Carbs 19, Protein 12

Eggplant Sandwich

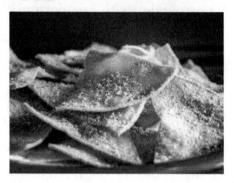

Preparation time: 5 minutes **Cooking time:** 30 minutes

Servings: 4

Ingredients:

- ✓ 1 tablespoon canola or sunflower oil
- ✓ medium whole-wheat tortillas
- ✓ ⅛ teaspoon coarse salt

Directions:

1 Preheat the oven to 350°F.

2 Brush the oil onto both sides of each tortilla. Stack them on a large cutting board, and cut the entire stack at once, cutting the stack into 8 wedges of each tortilla.

3 Transfer the tortilla pieces to a rimmed baking sheet. Sprinkle a little salt over each chip.

4 Bake for 10 minutes, and then flip the chips. Bake for another 3 to 5 minutes, until they're just starting to brown.

Nutrition:

Calories: 194 Total Fat: 11 g Saturated Fat: 2 g Cholesterol: 0 mg Sodium: 347 mg Carbohydrates: 20 g Fiber: 4 g Added Sugars: 0 g Protein: 4 g Potassium: 111 mg Vitamin K: 7 mcg

Cheese-Herb Dip

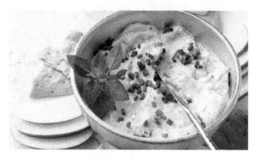

Preparation time: 20 minutes **Cooking time:** 0 minutes

Servings: 6

Ingredients:

- ✓ 1 cup Cream cheese
- ✓ ½ cup Unsweetened rice milk
- ✓ ½ Scallion
- ✓ 1 Tbsp Chopped fresh parsley
- ✓ 1 tbsp. Chopped fresh basil
- ✓ 1 tbsp Lemon juice
- ✓ 1 tsp Minced garlic
- ✓ ½ tsp Chopped fresh thyme
- ✓ ¼ tsp Ground black pepper

Directions:

1. In a bowl, mix the milk, cream cheese, parsley, scallion, basil, lemon juice, garlic, thyme, and pepper until well combined.
2. Store and use.

Nutrition:

Calories: 108 Fat: 10g Carb: 3g Phosphorus: 40mg Potassium: 52mg Sodium: 112mg Protein: 2g

Roasted Chili-Vinegar Peanuts

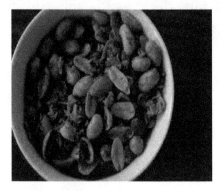

Preparation Time: 10 minutes **Cooking Time:** 5 minutes

Servings: 4

Ingredients:

- ✓ 1 tbsp. coconut oil
- ✓ 2 cups raw peanuts, unsalted
- ✓ 2 tsp. sea salt
- ✓ 1 tbsp. apple cider vinegar
- ✓ tsp. chili powder
- ✓ 1 tsp. fresh lime zest

Directions:

1 Preheat oven to 350°F.

2 In a large bowl, toss together the coconut oil, peanuts, and salt until well coated.

3 Transfer to a rimmed baking sheet and roast in the oven for about 15 minutes or until fragrant.

4 Transfer the roasted peanuts to a bowl and add vinegar,

chili powder, and lime zest.

5   Toss to coat well and serve.

Nutrition:

Calories: 447 Fats: 39.5 g Carbs: 12.3 g Protein: 18.9 g Sodium: 160 mg Potassium: 200 mg

Sweet and Spicy Kettle Corn

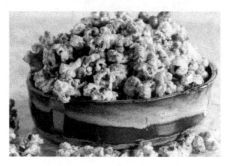

Preparation Time: 1 minute **Cooking Time:** 5 minutes

Servings: 8

Ingredients:

- ✓ 3 tbsp Olive oil
- ✓ cup Popcorn kernels
- ✓ ½ cup Brown sugar
- ✓ Pinch cayenne pepper

Directions:

1. Place a large pot with a lid over medium heat and add the olive oil with a few popcorn kernels.
2. Shake the pot lightly until the popcorn kernels pop. Add the rest of the kernels and sugar to the pot.
3. Pop the kernels with the lid on the pot, constantly shaking, until they are popped.
4. Remove the pot from the heat and transfer the popcorn to a large bowl.
5. Toss the popcorn with the cayenne pepper and serve.

Nutrition:

Calories: 186 Fat: 6g Carb: 30g Phosphorus: 85mg Potassium: 90mg Sodium: 5mg Protein: 3g

Baba Ghanoush

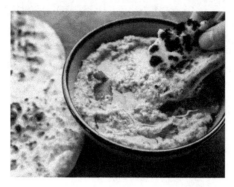

Preparation Time: 10 minutes **Cooking Time:** 1 hr 15 minutes

Servings: 8

Ingredients:

- ✓ 1 large eggplant, cut in half lengthwise
- ✓ 1 garlic head, unpeeled
- ✓ 2 tbsps. olive oil
- ✓ Lemon juice to taste

Directions:

1   Preheat the oven to 350°F.
2   Place the eggplant on the plate, skin-side up. Roast until the meat is very tender and detaches easily from the skin, about 1 hour depending on the eggplant's size. Let cool.
3   Meanwhile, cut the tip of the garlic cloves. Put garlic cloves in a square aluminum foil. Fold the edges of the

sheet and fold them together to form a tightly wrapped foil.

4   Roast with the eggplant until tender, about 20 minutes. Let cool. Purée the pods with a garlic press.

5   With a spoon, scoop out the eggplant's flesh and place it in the bowl of a food processor. Add the garlic purée, the oil, and the lemon juice. Stir until the purée is smooth.

6   Serve with mini pita bread.

Nutrition:

Calories: 110 Fats: 12 g Carbs: 5 g Protein: 1 g Sodium: 180 mg Potassium: 207 mg Phosphorus: 81 mg

Marinated Berries

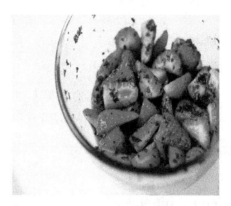

Preparation Time: 10 minutes **Cooking Time:** 30 minutes

Servings: 4

Ingredients:

- ✓ 2 cups fresh strawberries, hulled and quartered
- ✓ 1 cup fresh blueberries (optional)
- ✓ 2 tablespoons sugar
- ✓ 1 tablespoon balsamic vinegar
- ✓ 2 tablespons chopped fresh mint (optional)
- ✓ ⅛ teaspoon freshly ground black pepper

Directions:

1 Gently toss the strawberries, blueberries (if using), sugar, vinegar, mint (if using), and pepper in a large nonreactive bowl.

2 Let the flavors blend for at least 25 minutes, or as long as 2 hours.

Nutrition:

Calories: 73 Total Fat: 8 g Saturated Fat: 8 g Cholesterol: 0 mg Sodium: 4 mg Carbohydrates: 18 g Fiber: 2 g Added Sugars: 6 g Protein: 1 g Potassium: 162 mg Vitamin K: 9 mcg

Baked Pita Fries

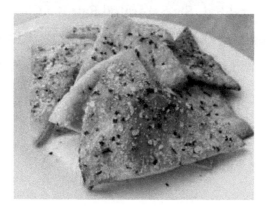

Preparation Time: 5 minutes **Cooking Time:** 15 minutes

Servings: 6

Ingredients:

- ✓ 3 pita loaves, 6 inches each
- ✓ 3 tbsps. olive oil
- ✓ Chili powder to taste

Directions:

1. Cut each bread in half with scissors to obtain 6 round pieces.
2. Cut each piece into eight points. Brush each with olive oil and sprinkle with chili powder.
3. Bake at 350°F for about 15 minutes until crisp.

Nutrition:

Calories:120 Fats:2.5 g Carbs:22 g Protein:3 g Sodium:70 mg

Thyme and Pineapple Crisp

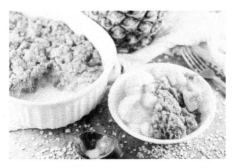

Preparation Time: 15 minutes **Cooking Time:** 15 minutes

Servings: 3

Ingredients:

- ✓ 1 can pineapple tidbits in juice, drained, reserving 1/3 cup juice
- ✓ ¼ cup brown sugar, divided
- ✓ 1 tablespoon cornstarch
- ✓ ½ teaspoon dried thyme leaves
- ✓ 3 tablespoons unsalted butter
- ✓ 1¼ cups quick-cooking oats
- ✓ 1/3 cup whole-wheat flour
- ✓ Pinch salt
- ✓ 1 tablespoon chopped walnuts

Directions:

1. Stir together the drained pineapple, reserved pineapple juice, One tablespoon brown sugar, cornstarch, and the thyme leaves in a saucepan over medium heat.

2 Cook for 8 to 10 minutes, the mixture is thickened. Meanwhile, combine the remaining Three tablespoons brown sugar and butter in a medium skillet over medium heat, frequently stirring, until the mixture melts.

3 Add the oats, flour, salt, and walnuts to the brown sugar mixture in the skillet.

4 Cook, frequently stirring, until the mixture is a deep golden brown, about 5 minutes. Transfer the oat mixture to a plate. When the pineapple mixture is thickened, top with the oatmeal mixture right in the saucepan and serve.

Nutrition:

Calories: 238; Total fat: 9g; Saturated fat: 4g; Sodium: 31mg; Potassium: 221mg; Phosphorus: 109mg; Carbohydrates: 39g; Fiber: 3g; Protein: 4g; Sugar: 20g

Happy Heart Energy Bites

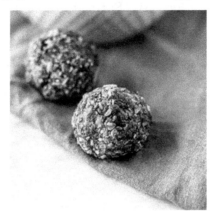

Preparation Time: 15 minutes **Cooking Time:** 30 minutes

Servings: 30

Ingredients:

- ✓ 1 cup rolled oats
- ✓ ¾ cup chopped walnuts
- ✓ ½ cup natural peanut butter
- ✓ ½ cup ground flaxseed
- ✓ ¼ cup honey
- ✓ ¼ cup dried cranberries

Directions:

1 Combine the oats, walnuts, peanut butter, flaxseed, honey, and cranberries in a large bowl.

2 Refrigerate for 10 to 20 minutes, if you can, to make them easier to roll.

3 Roll into ¾-inch balls. Store in the fridge or freezer.

Nutrition:

Calories: 174 Total Fat: 10 g Saturated Fat: 1 g Cholesterol: 0 mg Sodium: 43 mg Carbohydrates: 17 g Fiber: 3 g Added Sugars: 7 g Protein: 5 g Potassium: 169 mg Vitamin K: 1 mcg

Greek Cookies

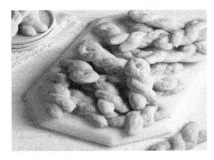

Preparation Time: 15 minutes **Cooking Time:** 1 hr 15 minutes

Servings: 6

Ingredients:

- ✓ ½ cup Plain yogurt
- ✓ ½ teaspoon baking powder
- ✓ 2 tablespoons Erythritol
- ✓ 1 teaspoon almond extract
- ✓ ½ teaspoon ground clove
- ✓ ½ teaspoon orange zest, grated
- ✓ tablespoons walnuts, chopped
- ✓ 1 cup wheat flour
- ✓ 1 teaspoon butter, softened
- ✓ 1 tablespoon honey
- ✓ tablespoons water

Directions:

1 In the mixing bowl mix up together Plain yogurt, baking

powder, Erythritol, almond extract, ground cloves orange zest, flour, and butter.

2 Knead the non-sticky dough. Add olive oil if the dough is very sticky and knead it well.

3 Then make the log from the dough and cut it into small pieces. Roll every piece of dough into the balls and transfer in the lined with baking paper tray.

4 Press the balls gently and bake for 25 minutes at 350F. Meanwhile, heat up together honey and water. Simmer the liquid for 1 minute and remove from the heat.

5 When the cookies are cooked, remove them from the oven and let them cool for 5 minutes.

6 Then pour the cookies with sweet honey water and sprinkle with walnuts.

7 Cool the cookies.

Nutrition:

Calories 134, Fat 3.4, Fiber 0.9, Carbs 26.1, Protein 4.3

Garlicky Cale Chips

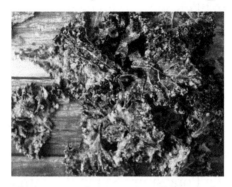

Preparation Time: 5 minutes **Cooking Time:** 25 minutes

Servings: 4

Ingredients:

- ✓ 1 bunch curly kale
- ✓ 2 teaspoons extra-virgin olive oil
- ✓ ¼ teaspoon kosher salt
- ✓ ¼ teaspoon garlic powder (optional)

Directions:

1 Preheat the oven to 325°F.

2 Remove the tough stems from the kale, and tear the leaves into squares about big potato chips (they'll shrink when cooked).

3 Transfer the kale to a large bowl, and drizzle with the oil. Massage with your fingers for 1 to 2 minutes to coat well. Spread out on the baking sheet.

4 Cook for 8 minutes, then toss and cook for another 7

minutes and check them. Take them out as soon as they feel crispy, likely within the next 5 minutes.

5   Sprinkle with salt and garlic powder (if using). Enjoy immediately.

Nutrition:

Calories: 28 Total Fat: 2 g Saturated Fat: 0 g Cholesterol: 0 mg Sodium: 126 mg Carbohydrates: 2 g Fiber: 1 g Added Sugars: 0 g Protein: 1 g Potassium: 81 mg Vitamin K: 114 mcg

Chicken-Vegetable Kebabs

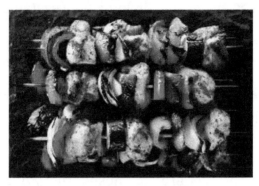

Preparation Time: 15 minutes **Cooking Time:** 20 minutes

Servings: 4

Ingredients:

- ✓ 2 tbsp Olive oil
- ✓ 2 tbsp. Freshly squeezed lemon juice
- ✓ ½ tsp Minced garlic
- ✓ ½ tsp Chopped fresh thyme
- ✓ 4 ounces Boneless, skinless chicken breast
- ✓ 1 Small summer squash
- ✓ ½ Medium onion

Directions:

1 Stir together the olive oil, lemon juice, garlic, and thyme in a bowl.

2 Add the chicken to the bowl and stir to coat.

3 Cover the bowl with plastic wrap and place the chicken in the refrigerator to marinate for 1 hour.

4   Thread the squash, onion, and chicken pieces onto four large skewers, evenly dividing the vegetable and meat among the skewers.

5   Heat a barbecue to medium and grill the skewers, turning at least two times, for 10 to 12 minutes or until the chicken is cooked through.

Nutrition:

Calories: 106 Fat: 8g Carb: 3g Phosphorus: 77mg Potassium: 199mg Sodium: 14mg Protein: 7g

Easy No-Bake Coconut Cookies

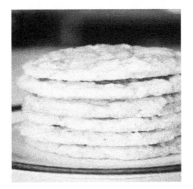

Preparation Time: 15 minutes **Cooking Time:** 20 minutes

Servings: 4

Ingredients:

- ✓ 3 cups coconut flakes, finely shredded
- ✓ 1 cup coconut oil, melted
- ✓ 1 tsp. liquid stevia

Directions:

1. Prepare all the ingredients in a large bowl, and stir until well blended.
2. Form the mixture into small balls and arrange them on a paper- lined baking tray.
3. Press each cookie down with a fork and refrigerate until firm. Enjoy!

Nutrition:

Calories: 99 Fats: 10 g Carbs: 2 g Protein: 3 g Sodium: 7 mg

Potassium: 105 mg Phosphorus: 11 mg

Dessert Recipes

Snickerdoodle Chickpea Blondies

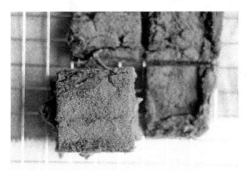

Preparation Time: 15 minutes **Cooking Time:** 30 minutes

Servings: 14

Ingredients:

- ✓ (15-oz.) can chickpeas, drained and rinsed
- ✓ 3 tbsps. nut butter of choice
- ✓ ¾ tsp. baking powder
- ✓ 2 tsps. vanilla extract
- ✓ 1/8 tsp. baking soda
- ✓ ¾ cup brown sugar
- ✓ 1 tbsp. applesauce, unsweetened
- ✓ ¼ cup ground flaxseed
- ✓ ¼ tsps. cinnamon

Directions:

1   Preheat the oven to 350°F. Grease an 8x8-inch baking pan. Blend all the ingredients in a food processor until very smooth. Scoop into the prepared baking pan.

2 Bake until the tops are medium golden brown, about 30–35 minutes.

Nutrition:

Calories: 85 Fats: 2 g Sodium: 7 mg Potassium: 62 mg Carbs: 16 g Fiber: 2 g Protein: 3 g

Tart Apple Granita

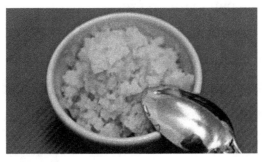

Preparation Time: 15 minutes **Cooking Time:** 0 minutes

Servings: 4

Ingredients:

- ✓ ½ cup granulated sugar
- ✓ ½ cup water
- ✓ 2 cups unsweetened apple juice
- ✓ ¼ cup freshly squeezed lemon juice

Directions:

1 In a small saucepan over medium-high heat, heat the sugar and water.

2 Bring the mixture to a boil and then reduce the heat to low and simmer for about 15 minutes or until the liquid has reduced by half.

3 Remove the pan from the heat and pour the liquid into a large shallow metal pan.

4 Let the liquid cool for about 30 minutes, and then stir

in the apple juice and lemon juice.

5   Place the pan in the freezer.

6   After 1 hour, run a fork through the liquid to break up any ice crystals formed. Scrape down the sides as well.

7   Place the pan back in the freezer and repeat the stirring and scraping every 20 minutes, creating slush.

8   Serve when the mixture is completely frozen and looks like crushed ice, after about 3 hours.

Nutrition:

Calories: 157 Fat: 0 g Carbohydrates: 0 g Phosphorus: 10 mg Potassium: 141 mg Sodium: 5 mg Protein: 0 g

Pot Chocolate Pudding Cake

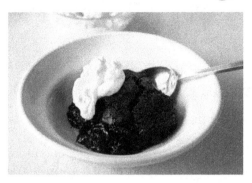

Preparation Time: 10 minutes **Cooking Time:** 4 minutes

Servings: 4

Ingredients:

- ✓ 2/3 cup chopped dark chocolate
- ✓ 1/2 cup applesauce
- ✓ 2 eggs
- ✓ 1 teaspoon vanilla
- ✓ 1/4 cup arrowroot
- ✓ 3 tablespoons cocoa
- ✓ powder powdered sugar for topping

Directions:

1. Start by pouring 2 cup water into the Instant pot and place trivet over it.
2. Add chocolate to a ramekin and place it over the trivet.
3. Switch the Instant pot to the Sauté mode and cook until the chocolate melts.

4 Whisk eggs, applesauce, and vanilla in a mixing bowl.

5 Stir in all the dry ingredients and mix well until fully incorporated.

6 Grease a 6-inch pan with butter and dust it with flour.

7 Spread the batter in the pan and place it in the Instant Pot. Seal the lid and cook for 4 minutes on Manual mode with High Pressure.

8 Once the cooking is done, release the pressure completely, then remove the pot's lid.

9 Allow the cake to cool, then remove it from the pan.

10 Slice and serve.

Nutrition:

Calories 210 Total Fats7 g Saturated Fat 4.5 g Cholesterol 23 mg Sodium 58 mg Total Carbs 35 g Fiber 1.0 g Sugar 2.9 g Protein 2 g

Blueberry Swirl Cake

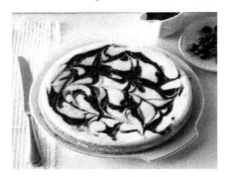

Preparation Time: 15 minutes **Cooking Time:** 45 minutes

Servings: 8

Ingredients:

- ✓ ½ cup margarine
- ✓ ¼ cups reduced-fat milk
- ✓ 1 cup granulated sugar
- ✓ 1 egg 1 egg white
- ✓ 1 tbsp. lemon zest, grated
- ✓ 1 tsp. cinnamon
- ✓ 1/3 cup light brown sugar
- ✓ ½ cups fresh blueberries
- ✓ ½ cups self-rising flour

Directions:

1   Cream the margarine and granulated sugar using an electric mixer at high speed until fluffy.

2   Add the egg and egg white and beat for another 2 minutes.

3   Add the lemon zest and reduce the speed to low.

4   Add the flour with milk alternately.

5   In a greased 13x19-inch pan, spread half of the batter and sprinkle with blueberry on top. Add the remaining batter.

6   Bake in a 350°F preheated oven for 45 minutes.

7   Let it cool on a wire rack before slicing and serving.

Nutrition:

Calories: 384 Carbs: 63 g Protein: 7 g Fats: 13 g
Phosphorus: 264 mg Potassium: 158 mg Sodium: 456 mg

Dessert Cocktail

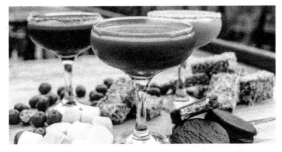

Preparation Time: 5 minutes **Cooking Time:** 0 minutes

Servings: 4

Ingredients:

- ✓ 1 cup of cranberry juice
- ✓ 1 cup of fresh ripe strawberries, washed and hull removed
- ✓ 2 tablespoon of lime juice
- ✓ ¼ cup of white sugar
- ✓ 8 ice cubes

Directions:

1 Combine all the ingredients in a blender until smooth and creamy.
2 Pour the liquid into tall chilled glasses and serve cold.

Nutrition:

Calories: 92 Carbohydrate: 23.5 g Protein: 0.5 g Sodium: 3.62 mg Potassium: 103.78 mg Phosphorus: 17.86 mg Dietary Fiber: 0.84 g Fat: 0.17 g

Peanut Butter Cookies

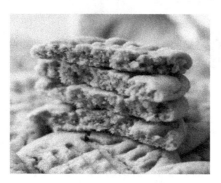

Preparation Time: 15 minutes **Cooking Time:** 25 minutes

Servings: 24

Ingredients:

- ✓ ¼ cup granulated sugar
- ✓ 1 cup unsalted peanut butter
- ✓ 1 tsp. baking soda
- ✓ 2 cups all-purpose flour
- ✓ 2 large eggs
- ✓ 2 tbsps. butter
- ✓ 2 tsps. pure vanilla extract
- ✓ 4 oz. softened cream cheese

Directions:

1 Line a cookie sheet with a non-stick liner. Set aside.
2 In a bowl, mix the flour, sugar, and baking soda. Set aside.
3 In a mixing bowl, combine the butter, cream cheese,

and peanut butter.

4 Mix on high speed until it forms a smooth consistency. Add the eggs and vanilla gradually while mixing until it forms a smooth consistency.

5 Add the almond flour mixture slowly and mix until well combined.

6 The dough is ready once it starts to stick together into a ball. Scoop the dough and drop each cookie on the prepared cookie sheet.

7 Press the cookie with a fork and bake for 10–12 minutes at 350°F.

Nutrition:

Calories: 138 Carbs: 12 g Protein: 4 g Fats: 9 g Phosphorus: 60 mg Potassium: 84 mg Sodium: 31 mg

Pumpkin Chocolate Cake

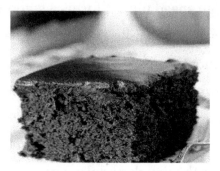

Preparation Time: 10 minutes **Cooking Time:** 25 minutes

Servings: 6

Ingredients:

- ✓ 2 cups flour
- ✓ 1 tablespoon pumpkin pie spice
- ✓ 1 teaspoon baking soda
- ✓ Two sticks- 1 cup unsalted butter, softened
- ✓ 1-1/4 cup sugar
- ✓ 1 egg
- ✓ 2 teaspoons vanilla extract
- ✓ 1 cup cream cheese
- ✓ 1 package 12 oz. chocolate chips

Directions:

1 Whisk pumpkin pie spice, flour, and baking soda in a mixing bowl.

2 Beat sugar with butter in a mixer until fluffy.

3 Whisk in egg, vanilla, and cream cheese.

196

4   Beat well, then gradually add the flour mixture while mixing continuously.

5   Fold in the chocolate chips and grease 2 Bundt pans with cooking oil.

6   Divide the batter into the pans and cover them with aluminum foil.

7   Pour 1.5 cups of water into the Instant Pot and place rack over it.

8   Set one Bundt on the rack and seal the lid.

9   Cook for 20 minutes on Manual mode with High pressure. Once done, release the pressure completely, then remove the lid.

10 Cook the other cake in the Bundt pan following the same method.

11 Allow the cakes to cool, then slice to serve.

Nutrition:

Calories 232 Total Fats11 g Saturated Fat 6.5 g Cholesterol 7 mg Sodium 112 mg Total Carbs 30 g Fiber 0.4 g Sugar 0.5 g Protein 3 g

Vanilla Custard

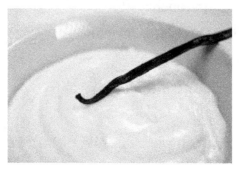

Preparation Time: 10 minutes **Cooking Time:** 10 minutes

Servings: 8

Ingredients:

- ✓ 1 Egg
- ✓ 1/8 tsp Vanilla
- ✓ 1/8 tsp Nutmeg
- ✓ ½ cup Almond milk
- ✓ 2 Tbsp Stevia

Directions:

1 Scald the milk, then let it cool slightly.

2 Break the egg into a bowl and beat it with the nutmeg.

3 Add the scalded milk, the vanilla, and the sweetener to taste. Mix well.

4 Place the bowl in a baking pan filled with ½ deep of water. Bake for 30 minutes at 325F.

5 Serve.

Nutrition:

Calories: 167.3 Fat: 9 g Carbs: 11 g Phosphorus: 205 mg
Potassium: 249 mg Sodium: 124 mg Protein: 10 g

Mixed Berry Cobbler

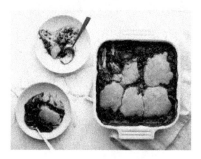

Preparation Time: 10 minutes **Cooking Time:** 4 hr

Servings: 8

Ingredients:

- ✓ ¼ cup coconut milk
- ✓ ¼ cup ghee
- ✓ ¼ cup honey
- ✓ ½ cup almond flour
- ✓ ½ cup tapioca starch
- ✓ ½ tbsp. cinnamon
- ✓ ½ tbsp. coconut sugar
- ✓ 1 tsp. vanilla
- ✓ 12 oz. raspberries, frozen
- ✓ 16 oz. wild blueberries, frozen
- ✓ 2 tsps. baking powder
- ✓ 2 tsps. tapioca starch

Directions:

1 Place the frozen berries in the slow cooker. Add the

honey and 2 tsp. tapioca starch. Mix to combine.

2   In a bowl, mix the tapioca starch, almond flour, coconut milk, ghee, baking powder, and vanilla. Sweeten with the sugar. Place this pastry mix on top of the berries.

3   Cook in the slow cooker for 4 hours.

Nutrition:

Calories: 146 Carbs: 33 g Protein: 1 g Fats: 3 g Phosphorus: 29 mg Potassium: 133 mg Sodium: 4 mg

Almond Butter Mousse

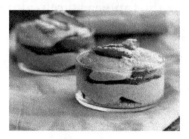

Preparation Time: 10 minutes **Cooking Time:** 7 minutes

Servings: 3

Ingredients:

- ✓ 2 strawberries
- ✓ 1 cup coconut milk
- ✓ ½ tsp. vanilla extract
- ✓ 2 tsps. erythritol
- ✓ 4 tbsps. almond butter
- ✓ ¾ tsp. ground cinnamon

Directions:

1 Pour the coconut milk into the food processor.
2 Add vanilla extract, erythritol, almond butter, and ground cinnamon.
3 Blend the mixture until smooth.
4 Ten transfer it in the saucepan and start to preheat it over medium heat.
5 Stir it all the time.
6 When the mousse starts to be thick, remove it from the

heat and stir.

7 Pour the mousse into the serving glasses.

8 Slice the strawberries.

9 Top the mousse with the strawberries.

Nutrition:

Calories: 321 g Fats: 31.1 g Fiber: 4.4 g Carbs: 9.6 g Protein:
6.4 g

Almond Butter Mousse

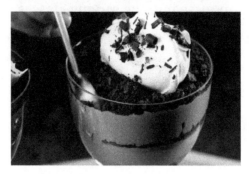

Preparation Time: 2 hr **Cooking Time:** 0 minutes

Servings: 4

Ingredients:

- ✓ 2 tablespoons cocoa powder
- ✓ 1 cup almond milk
- ✓ 1 tablespoon chia seeds
- ✓ Pinch of salt
- ✓ ½ teaspoon vanilla extract

Directions:

1 Take a bowl and add cocoa powder, almond milk, chia seeds, vanilla extract, and stir.

2 Transfer to dessert glass and place in your fridge for 2 hours.

3 Serve and enjoy!

Nutrition:

Calories: 130 Fat: 5 g Carbohydrates: 7 g Protein: 16 g

Almond Truffles

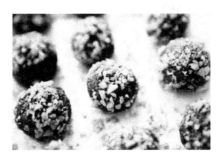

Preparation Time: 20 minutes **Cooking Time:** 5 minutes

Servings: 5

Ingredients:

- ✓ ½ cup almond flour
- ✓ 2 tsps. almond butter
- ✓ ¾ tsp. ground cinnamon
- ✓ 1 tsp. liquid Stevia
- ✓ 1 oz. dark chocolate
- ✓ 1 tbsp. heavy cream

Directions:

1 Mix up together the almond flour and almond butter.

2 Add the ground cinnamon and liquid Stevia®.

3 Mix up the mixture until smooth.

4 Then make 5 truffles and place them on the baking paper. Freeze them for 15 minutes in the freezer.

5 Meanwhile, preheat the dark chocolate and heavy cream. When the mixture is homogenous, the chocolate

batter is cooked.

6   Remove the truffles from the freezer and sprinkle them with the chocolate batter.

7   Let the cooked truffles chill.

Nutrition:

Calories: 98 Fats: 8.1 g Fiber: 1.5 g Carbs: 5.4 g Protein: 2.2 g

Vanilla Biscuits

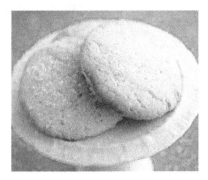

Preparation Time: 20 minutes **Cooking Time:** 40 minutes

Servings: 1

Ingredients:

- ✓ 5 eggs
- ✓ ½ cup coconut flour
- ✓ ½ cup wheat flour
- ✓ 1 teaspoon vanilla extract
- ✓ Cooking spray

Directions:

1 Crack the eggs in the mixing bowl and mix it up with the help of the hand mixer.

2 Then add wheat flour, coconut flour, and vanilla extract.

3 Mix it for 30 seconds.

4 Spray the baking tray with cooking spray.

5 Pour the biscuit mixture into the tray and flatten it.

6 Bake it for 40 minutes at 3500 F.

7 When the biscuit is cooked, cut it into squares and serve.

Nutrition:

Calories 132; Fat 4.7; Fiber 4.3; Phosphorus: 21mg; Potassium: 145mg; Sodium: 20mg; Carbs 28.3; Protein 7

Carrot Cake

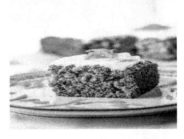

Preparation Time: 20 minutes **Cooking Time:** 50 minutes

Servings: 6

Ingredients:

- ✓ ½ cups whole wheat pastry flour
- ✓ 3/4 teaspoons baking powder
- ✓ 3/4 teaspoons baking soda
- ✓ ½ teaspoons ground cinnamon
- ✓ ¼ teaspoons ground cardamom
- ✓ ¼ teaspoons ground allspice
- ✓ ¼ teaspoons ground ginger

Wet Cake Ingredients:

- ✓ tablespoons ground flaxseed, mixed with ¼ cup warm water ½ cup almond milk
- ✓ ½ teaspoons orange flower water, or substitute vanilla

Cake Mix in Ingredients:

- ✓ 1 cup shredded carrot

Icing Ingredients:

- ✓ ½ cup cashews
- ✓ ½ cup water, plus more as needed
- ✓ ½ teaspoons orange flower water

Directions:

1. Start by adding 1.5 cups of water into Instant Pot and place a trivet over it.
2. Grease a pan with cooking oil, suitable to fit the Instant Pot.
3. Prepare the batter by mixing the dry and wet ingredients separately.
4. Now mix the two mixtures in a large bowl.
5. Spread this batter in the prepared, and then cover it with aluminum foil.
6. Place the pan in the Instant Pot and seal its lid.
7. Cook for 50 minutes on "Manual" mode with high pressure. Meanwhile, prepare the icing by cooking cashews, date, and water in a saucepan to boil.
8. Allow it to cool, then blend this mixture in a blender until smooth.
9. Spread this icing over the baked cake.

Nutrition:

Calories: 184 Total Fats: 9 g Saturated Fat: 4.5 g Cholesterol: 0 mg Sodium: 94 mg Total Carbs: 22 g Fiber: 8 g Sugar: 0.8 g Protein: 4 g

Fragrant Lava Cake

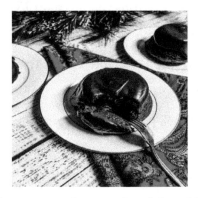

Preparation Time: 20 minutes **Cooking Time:** 20 minutes

Servings: 6

Ingredients:

- ✓ 1 tsp. vanilla extract
- ✓ 2 eggs, whisked
- ✓ 4 tbsps. cocoa powder
- ✓ 2 tbsps. erythritol
- ✓ 8 tbsps. heavy cream
- ✓ 4 tsps. almond flour
- ✓ Cooking spray

Directions:

1 Whisk the eggs together with heavy cream.
2 Then add the vanilla extract, erythritol, cocoa powder, and almond flour.
3 Mix the mixture until smooth.
4 Spray the mini cake molds with the cooking spray.

5   Preheat the oven to 350°F.

6   Pour the cake mix into the cake molds and place in the oven. Bake the cakes for 15 minutes.

7   Then remove the lava cakes from the oven and from the cake molds.

8   Serve the lava cakes only hot.

Nutrition:

Calories:218 g Fats:19.1 g Fiber:3.7 g Carbs:8.3 g Protein:8.1 g

CPSIA information can be obtained
at www.ICGtesting.com
Printed in the USA
BVHW061929220321
603177BV00010B/624

9 781914 025785